GENDERED BODIES AND LEISURE

With its roots in Middle Eastern and North African dance, belly dance is a popular leisure activity in the West with women (and some men) of all ages and body types pursuing the activity for diverse reasons. Drawing on empirical research, fieldwork, and interviews with participants, this book investigates the social world and small group cultures of American belly dance, examining the various ways in which people use leisure to construct the self and social relationships.

With attention to gender expectations, body image, sexuality, community, spiritual experiences, and the process of identifying with a leisure activity, this book shows how people engage in the same pursuit in a variety of ways. It sheds light on the manner in which dancers strive to deal with the challenges presented by internal power struggles and legitimacy bids, public beliefs, narrow cultural ideals of beauty, and often sexualized assumptions about their art.

A fascinating study of identity work and the reproduction and challenging of gender norms through a gendered leisure activity, *Gendered Bodies and Leisure: The practice and performance of American belly dance* will be of interest to students and scholars researching gender and sexuality, the sociology of leisure, the sociology of the body, and interactionist thought.

Rachel Kraus is Professor of Sociology at Ball State University, USA.

Interactionist Currents

Series editors:
Dennis Waskul, Minnesota State University, USA
Simon Gottschalk, University of Nevada Las Vegas, USA

Interactionist Currents publishes contemporary interactionist works of exceptional quality to advance the state of symbolic interactionism. Rather than revisiting classical symbolic interactionist or pragmatist theory, however, this series extends the boundaries of interactionism by examining new empirical topics in subject areas that interactionists have not sufficiently examined; systematizing, organizing, and reflecting on the state of interactionist knowledge in subfields both central and novel within interactionist research; connecting interactionism with contemporary intellectual movements; and illustrating the contemporary relevance of interactionism in ways that are interesting, original, and enjoyable to read.

Recognizing an honored and widely appreciated theoretical tradition, reflecting on its limitations, and opening new opportunities for the articulation of related perspectives and research agendas, this series presents work from across the social sciences that makes explicit use of interactionist ideas and concepts, interactionist research, and interactionist theory – both classical and contemporary.

Titles in this series

Challenging Myths of Masculinity
Michael Atkinson & Lee F. Monaghan
ISBN: 978-1-4094-3500-6

The Drama of Social Life
Edited by Charles Edgley
ISBN: 978-1-4094-5190-7

The Politics of Sorrow
Daniel D. Martin
ISBN: 978-1-4094-4634-7

Gendered Bodies and Leisure
The practice and performance of American belly dance

RACHEL KRAUS

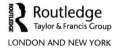

Routledge
Taylor & Francis Group

LONDON AND NEW YORK

First published 2017
by Routledge
2 Park Square, Milton Park, Abingdon, Oxon OX14 4RN

and by Routledge
711 Third Avenue, New York, NY 10017

Routledge is an imprint of the Taylor & Francis Group, an informa business

© 2017 Rachel Kraus

British Library Cataloguing in Publication Data
A catalogue record for this book is available from the British Library

Library of Congress Cataloguing in Publication Data
Names: Kraus, Rachel, author.
Title: Gendered bodies and leisure: the practice and
performance of American belly dance / Rachel Kraus.
Description: Milton Park, Abingdon, Oxon; New York, NY:
Routledge, 2016. | Includes bibliographical references and index.
Identifiers: LCCN 2016005962 | ISBN 9781472419736 (hardback) |
ISBN 9781315569024 (ebook)
Subjects: LCSH: Belly dance–United States.
Classification: LCC GV1798.5. K73 2016 | DDC 793.3–dc23
LC record available at http://lccn.loc.gov/2016005962

ISBN: 978-1-4724-1973-6 (hbk)
ISBN: 978-1-3155-6902-4 (ebk)

Typeset in Bembo
by Out of House Publishing

Contents

List of figures

Acknowledgments

I am exceedingly grateful to many individuals, groups, and organizations for their invaluable contributions to this project. First and foremost, this endeavor would not be possible without the participation of the many dancers (current and former) who graciously took time out of their very busy schedules to share their stories with me. I sincerely appreciate their insights, thoughtful reflections, and openness. Our conversations and interactions form the backbone of this book.

I also want to acknowledge my many dance instructors, workshop leaders, and troupe directors over the years who taught me about innumerable aspects of the belly dance world, including history, styles, language, and norms. These very helpful mentors include Carenza bint Asya, Celeste (Isabelle Murray), Stacy DuVall, Kate Greenwalt Huber, Jeana Jorgensen, Kat Lebo, and Liz Wray. I am grateful to all of my fellow dancers, current and former troupe mates, drummers, musicians, and various audience members who have greatly contributed to my experiences with belly dance and inform many of the insights presented within these pages. Angie Andriot, Kat Lebo, and Kelly Marshall Riddle provided some very helpful feedback on earlier drafts of this manuscript. I very much appreciate their candor and perspectives from inside the belly dance world.

Furthermore, I wish to thank the past and present members of the Ball State Belly Dance Club, especially the founding officers, Caitlin Matchett, Jessica Matchett, Rachel Penticuff, and Ashley Schuyler. I also appreciate the hard work of the club presidents over the years, including Andrea Harmon, Bridget Hartman, and Miranda Martin. I also appreciate Jackie Jones-Sowinski and Jenny Smithson for assisting the club with lessons, practices, and events. In my position as faculty advisor, I have greatly enjoyed working with everyone involved with the club and our time together has given me yet additional insight into the world of belly dance.

Monetary support for this project was supplied by a few institutions. I was awarded a New Faculty Research Grant at Ball State University, which allowed me to conduct the first set of interviews. The Association for the Sociology of Religion provided a Fichter Research Grant that supported the second set of interviews and helped cover transcription costs. The research for this book would not have been possible without the support of these funds.

Of course I thank my academic institution, Ball State University in Muncie, Indiana where I have worked since 2005. I deeply appreciate the intellectual freedom and creativity that I have been afforded there. I am especially grateful for the continuing support from my department Chairs, Melinda Messineo and Roger Wojtkiewicz, and faculty in the sociology department. They have encouraged me throughout this project and supported me in many ways.

I have been encouraged and assisted by many colleagues, professionals, and friends. Over the years, several scholars have read drafts of various papers that have contributed to the material in this book. They include, but are not limited to, Michele Dillon, Rachel L. Einwohner, Mellisa Holtzman, Amy Petts, Richard J. Petts, David Yamane, and various anonymous reviewers. This project has also greatly benefited from conversations with Rev. Bob Hunter, Carolyn A. Kapinus, Charis E. Kubrin, Angela M. Moe, Lisa Pellerin, J. William Spencer, and William Swatos. I am also grateful to Drs. Rhadika Walling and Irene Fox and Judith Villegas who have helped keep me healthy throughout this project. Furthermore, I appreciate constant reminders from my childhood friend, Joanna Jones, about how good I would feel when this book is finished (and she is right).

This project has benefited greatly from the work of numerous research assistants. These individuals have helped with interview transcription, data entry, literature searches, and reference formatting. I sincerely appreciate the work of Ashley Brooke Baker, Brendan J. L. Dugan, Daniel R. Flowers, R. David Frantzreb II, Pooja Naidu, Morgan Roddy, Jared Sell, and Amanda Zimmerman for their very helpful research assistance.

I appreciate the patience of many undergraduate and graduate students at Ball State who have sat through my classes while I talked with them about belly dance. Sharing connections between studying belly dance and the course material I teach in numerous classes, including gender, social psychology, and research methods helped me flush out several ideas presented in these pages. Furthermore, my students asked insightful questions and commented on the information I shared with them, which pushed me to further explore my thoughts.

I am extraordinarily grateful to the publishers, editors, and reviewers at Ashgate with whom it has been an absolute pleasure to work. I was privileged to work with outstanding editors, Dennis Waskul, Phillip Vannini, and Simon Gottschalk who offered extremely helpful suggestions on numerous drafts of various chapters. Dennis provided key analytic suggestions on several chapters and never hesitated to respond to my plethora of email inquiries. Neil Jordan was invaluable for helping me navigate the logistics of book publishing. I am grateful to two anonymous reviewers who provided insightful feedback and suggestions on an earlier draft of this book.

I appreciate several people's assistance with photographs. I am grateful to the restaurant and shop owners who allowed me to photograph inside their businesses. I sincerely appreciate Carrie Meyer at The Dancers Eye (www. thedancerseye.com) who donated some of her beautiful pictures to this book.

As I reflect on the process of writing this book and the many years I have spent involved in and formally studying the world of belly dance, my greatest debt is to my family. My mother, Ruth Kraus, frequently inquired about the book and supported my involvement in belly dance from early on. The very first conversation I had with anyone about this project was with my husband, Scott A. Desmond, as we sat around a table at Mountain Jacks, a restaurant in Lafayette, Indiana. Over the years, we have had countless talks about this research resulting in a myriad of insights and perspectives. He has stood by me through my most frustrating and sad moments in addition to sharing exciting and uplifting experiences. He accompanied me on several belly dance outings and his viewpoints on events provided meaningful insights into many aspects of belly dance. Most importantly, Scott's unwavering support and encouragement was crucial for the completion of this book. Finally, I appreciate Buster's (our Yorkie) non-human type of support who sat next to me on the couch while I typed and was kind enough to provide occasional breaks with his barking at random noises, passersby, and the occasional other dog.

Portions of the material in Chapter 5 can be found in the following articles:

Kraus, Rachel. 2009. "Straddling the Sacred and Secular: Creating a Spiritual Experience through Belly Dance." *Sociological Spectrum* 29(5):598–625.
Kraus, Rachel. 2014. "Transforming Spirituality in Artistic Leisure: How the Spiritual Meaning of Belly Dance Changes over Time." *Journal for the Scientific Study of Religion* 53(3):459–478.

Portions of the material in Chapter 8 can be found in the following article:

Kraus, Rachel. 2010. "We are not Strippers": How Belly Dancers Manage a (Soft) Stigmatized Serious Leisure Activity." *Symbolic Interaction* 33(3): 435–455.

Chapter 1

The social world of belly dance

In August 2002, I return to graduate school after nine months of conducting fieldwork in Washington, D.C. for my dissertation. I have taken yoga classes at a nearby recreation center and am eager to participate in another physical activity. Browsing through the center's catalogue, I find a listing for belly dance classes. I have always enjoyed the arts, I like to dance, and belly dance sounded exotic and different to me. I register for an introductory class that I assume will be an enjoyable way to meet people, get some exercise, and dance. However, I soon learn that belly dance is multi-dimensional. I am struck by the backgrounds of the people in my classes. They are primarily graduate students or professionals in fields such as biology, chemistry, math, law, the military, and pharmacy. I and only a few other women are involved in the social sciences. Almost all of the participants are female, and I am amazed by the variety of ages (college freshman to women approaching retirement) and bodies (short, petite, tall, and voluptuous) of the people in my dance class.

I clearly am not in a typical fitness program where I might expect the participants to be primarily younger and thinner. Furthermore, unlike many aerobics classes, belly dance does not stop when the class ends. I eventually learn that dancers gather together on weekends to listen and dance to music, participate in public belly dance performances, attend instructional dance workshops, and design costumes. I began to think about belly dance as not only a class that I visit once a week, but a social world with norms, values, beliefs, rewards, and challenges. I want to take a closer look at this world and the subculture surrounding it.

This book draws from over thirteen years of my personal experience in various belly dance communities. I've taken weekly classes and intensive workshops since 2002. During this time, I've also been a member of two student and one professional troupe. Along with my autoethnographic experiences, I conducted over 120 formal interviews (about a third of which are multiple conversations with the same dancers over a five-year period) and participated in numerous informal interactions. Approaching belly dance from a sociological perspective, I focus on social aspects of the activity more than historical or artistic components of the dance. Specifically, I examine belly dance as a female-dominated adult subculture that surrounds sustained involvement in a leisure activity.

Belly dance is an intriguing pursuit to examine because it provides insight into a leisure subculture dominated by adult women of all ages, while also attracting a sprinkling of men. Leisure activities and subcultures are sites for identity construction and gender projects (Green 1998; Wilkins 2008). Yet, much of the existing scholarly work focuses on youth, young adults, males, gamers, and music (Anderson and Taylor 2010; Fine 2002; Jones 2000; Haenfler 2006, 2010; Hunt 2004; Hunt 2008; Wilkins 2008). Studies of riot grrrls (Haenfler 2010) and girls' "bedroom culture" (McRobbie and Garber 1976) are notable exceptions that examine various girl subcultures, but even studies such as these focus on youth. Investigating belly dance sheds light on how adult women and men use leisure and subcultural symbols for the construction of the self and social relationships, how participants manage interactions with (sometimes skeptical and hostile) outsiders, and how gender norms are reproduced and resisted. Specifically, belly dance is a site where global culture mixes with colonized appropriations, sexuality is highly contested and heavily monitored, rhetoric about women's empowerment and body acceptance are used to protest narrow Western cultural ideals, and men navigate a minority status.

In this book, I highlight belly dance in the United States. My focus on American dancers is not meant to ignore the very significant and meaningful presence of belly dance throughout the world, especially in its original cultures of the Middle East and North Africa. As the constructed meaning of belly dance and the role it plays in different societies inevitably varies, I situate belly dance within an American context because many dancers' experiences are direct responses to American culture. Furthermore, Shay (2008) argues that American women use belly dance for identity construction. In the midst of a culture where "whiteness" is associated with normalcy and being non-white provides a more salient identity (Wilkins 2008), belly dance participants borrow non-Western cultural tools to create an "exotic" component of the self. Because one of the primary goals of this book is to examine how people use leisure to negotiate their identities, American belly dance is a well-suited site for investigation.

Behind belly dance

Belly dance is a dance form that consists of isolations, undulations, and shimmies that are primarily executed using the center of the body, hips, chest, and shoulders (Al-Rawi 1999; Shay and Sellers-Young 2005). In belly dance, shimmies refer to rapid up and down or forward and backward movements of the hips or shoulders. Undulations are best described as body waves where the chest moves forward, up, drops back, and returns to a neutral position.

2

Isolations involve areas of the body moving individually and independently from one another; one or a few body parts are in motion, while others are still. Along with shimmies, isolations, and undulations, basic movements include hip bumps (imagine that your arms are full, so you need to close your car door with your hip). Sliding the head, hips, and chest from side to side are additional common moves. The arms and legs are primarily used to frame movements originating from the body's core (AlZayer 2004; Dox 2006; Sellers-Young 1992; Shay and Sellers-Young 2005).

Many belly dance scholars and writers suggest that the activity is one of the oldest dance forms in the world dating back to between 3,000 and 25,000 BCE (Al-Rawi 1999; Hobin 2003; Sharif 2004). Although its precise roots are difficult to ascertain, it is widely accepted within belly dance communities that the dance is based on solo and improvisational ancient folk and social dances from North African and Middle Eastern countries, particularly Egypt and Turkey (Al Zayer 2004; Dox 2006; Hobin 2003; Shay and Sellers-Young 2005). Some scholars and dancers argue that these dances have been part of fertility and life-cycle celebrations, funerals, social gatherings, and religious rituals to connect with the divine (Hobin 2003; Sellers-Young 1992; Sharif 2004).

Today, belly dance (often referred to by other names that I will discuss shortly) continues to be practiced both privately and publicly in its countries of origin. Despite its reputation as a somewhat lowly form of entertainment, belly dance is popular and is performed publicly by professional dancers at restaurants, weddings, and other celebrations (Shay 2008). Privately, women and men (but not always together) dance as a creative, relaxing, and social pastime to entertain themselves and guests in their homes (Al Zayer 2004; Sellers-Young 1992; Sharif 2004). In its countries of origins, belly dance is comparable to the social dancing observed in American bars, clubs, festivals, or weddings. The style of dancing is meant for entertainment, but not considered a promising or highly respected career path.

Although the origins of belly dance are based in community and social dances with fairly utilitarian purposes, in the United States the dance consists of polished movements that are combined with Westernized costumes and used to entertain various publics. Many participants view the activity as a studio-taught cultural and artistic dance form worthy of dedicated and intense formal instruction. Teachers emphasize proper posture, technique, and stage presence (Dox 2006; Rees-Denis 2008). Both women and men take regular classes and intense instructional workshops to learn various belly dance movements, choreographies, and styles (Carlton 1994; Sellers-Young 1992). In fact, it is difficult today to find a city in the United States that does not offer belly dance instruction at a recreation center, fitness club, college, or studio (Belly Dance Classes in the United States 2014).

Belly dance as artistic leisure

"Dance is art," Lana, an instructor of several decades tells me. She continues to describe belly dance as:

> An improvisational art form, which makes it different from many other dance forms. Historically speaking we work with live music, so it's the perfect melting of the dance, art, and music because our bodies are the instruments. The musician may play his instrument, but with oriental dance, it is an improvisational art form. You join with the musicians. You become one with the musicians. Your body becomes the instrument. So, it's sublime. It is art in the moment.

Like some other artistic dance forms, such as ballroom (Marion 2008), belly dance consists of multiple components, primarily the artist and audience. As Lana implies, musicians also play an important role. Music provides rhythms for bodily movements which, in turn, highlight and accentuate the tunes (DeNora 2000; Stephens and Delamont 2006). Similar to staging opera performances to follow the music (Atkinson 2006), some belly dance moves, such as hip bumps, lifts, and drops, shimmies, and various arm movements accentuate musical notes to emphasize down beats or particular climactic points in the music. In belly dance, we refer to creatively and effectively matching movements to musical bars as musicality.

Andy, a dancer with over thirty-five years of experience, tells me that belly dance is an art form because "it takes a lot of study to do it correctly." Speaking about the Belly Dance Superstars (a professional international touring group of belly dancers), he says, "All the dancers are really highly trained. A lot of people think you stand there and wiggle your hips or shake your arms. But, it really takes a lot of training." Producing art requires collaboration among artists (Becker 2001). As Andy alludes to, and much like ballroom dance (Marion 2008), a large part of this collaboration occurs between instructors and students. Participants do not learn belly dance in a vacuum. They take regular lessons, such as weekly classes, and more intensive workshops in a variety of settings, such as studios or fitness facilities. Dance students also learn from books and videos.

Along with constructing belly dance as an art form, the activity constitutes a type of leisure for many participants in the United States. Leisure refers to a voluntary pastime people pursue with a positive state of mind (Stebbins 2011). Because it is an elective way to spend free time, and not a primary source of income, people more easily move in and out of a leisure pursuit compared to paid work on which people depend for their livelihoods (Stebbins 2001). Although several dancers who were prominent in the beginning of the twentieth century made good careers out of performing belly dance (Shay 2008), most people involved in belly dance today do not earn a living through the activity. However, some dancers are occasionally paid for a performance and/or earn supplemental income through teaching classes and/or workshops.

Belly dancers frequently perform in a variety of public settings, such as international events, art and renaissance festivals, farmers' markets, and a host of restaurants and clubs. They are also involved in a variety of charitable causes and educational projects, dancing at libraries, schools, hospitals, nursing homes, and various fundraisers (Dox 2006). On a smaller scale, a belly dancer may be hired to dance at corporate events or private parties celebrating birthdays and anniversaries.

Because it is more of a leisure activity than a livelihood for the vast majority of dancers, in some ways, people "pay to play" in this social world. Much like ballroom dancers who spend thousands of dollars on costumes, shoes, and jewelry (Marion 2008), belly dancers purchase skirts, pants, tops, decorated bras, vests, coats, belts, scarves, jewelry, and props. Full costumes for women, which may consist of a dress or a two-piece top and skirt ensemble, can range from $100 to $700. A hip scarf or belt can cost between $30 and $90. Depending on the quality of the set, zills range in price from $5 to $50 for two finger cymbals. Belly dancers sometimes dance with swords, baskets, fans, or veils as props, which can cost between $20 and $200. Dancers spend money on weekly classes and intensive workshops. Weekly classes range from $10 to $15 per one-hour session. Private one-hour lessons may range from $25 to $50 or more. Depending on the instructor, workshops may cost around $40–$90 per two-hour session. Although belly dance can be a significant financial investment, participants spend money to different degrees, so dancers from a variety of social class backgrounds participate in belly dance. For instance, some only take weekly classes and never take a workshop. Some dancers acquire minimal costume pieces and/or make their own, while others purchase dozens of skirts, tops, and jewelry pieces. For instance, in the summer of 2015, I own three skirts suitable for performance. A few women in my dance troupe own hanging organizers jammed with around twenty skirts. The significant financial investment that many people make in belly dance has consequences for interactions and relationships between dancers that I will discuss in the coming chapters.

The controversial label of "belly dance"

The term "belly dance" is highly debatable among many people who participate in this activity. Some people question whether modern-day belly dance in the United States accurately portrays dancing from its Middle Eastern and North African countries of origin (Sellers-Young 1992; Shay 2008). It is not my intention to argue what movements, styles, and costumes truly count as belly dance. I will leave to the dancers and other scholars to determine the accuracy and authenticity of belly dance for themselves. Rather, I explore the social world of belly dance, highlighting how women and men use cultural resources within leisure subcultures to construct their identities and social relationships.

The Middle East and North Africa are occasionally collectively referred to as "the Orient," so belly dance is sometimes called "Oriental dance." In the Middle East, belly dance is known as "Raqs Sharqi" or "Raks el Sharki," which in English translates into "dance of the East" or "Middle Eastern dance." "Belly dance" comes from the French term "Danse du Ventre" (abdominal dance), and was used to describe some of the first public performances in the United States (Carlton 1994; Monty 1986). To varying degrees, some dancers distinguish between "belly dance" and "Middle Eastern" dance (or any other of the aforementioned names), and some of these differences will be illuminated throughout this book.

I use the term "belly dance" because I focus on American dancers. Also, the dance styles discussed in this book include Western adaptations of more traditional Middle Eastern dance, such as American Tribal Style, American cabaret, and tribal fusion (which brings together a variety of dance forms and music styles). Furthermore, I believe the term "belly dance" is a more well-known linguistic anchor with which a broader audience is familiar. Finally, I opt not to use "Middle Eastern" dance because this term sometimes refers to dances not covered in this book, such as Iranian, Japanese, and Indian classical dance (Shay 2008).

The varieties of belly dance

Belly dance is not a single style of dance. It is a continuously evolving mixture of cultures, movements, and styles. Similar to several types of ballroom dance (Marion 2008), there are various dance styles that fall under the broad category of belly dance. Each of these styles has norms and guidelines regarding movements, costuming, and music. There are also pioneers who are deemed authorities on each type of dance and are credited with creating and disseminating the dance. Although each style has some defining qualities and characteristics, dancers frequently combine genres with one another and create their own form.

Although there are variations, belly dancers share some common costuming practices. To varying degrees, costumes for female dancers emphasize traditionally feminine features of the body, such as the breasts and hips. Most styles of belly dance include some type of belt and/or scarf worn around the hips,

6

skirts and/or pants, bras or tops covering the chest to varying degrees, some form of makeup, and carefully styled hair. Men's costumes tend to consist of harem pants and vests that cover the torso to varying degrees and/or light shirts. Some men wrap their hair in turbans. Group-specific clothing, such as costumes, have meaning within the communities of which they are a part (Connell 2002). Like the different styles and costumes within ballroom dance that mark group membership (Marion 2008), belly dance costumes, in part, signify one's particular dance style and group affiliation.

American cabaret, sometimes referred to as nightclub, is the glamorous, show business style that most people probably associate with belly dance. The cabaret style developed in the 1920s in Middle Eastern nightclubs possibly to cater to the tastes of travelers from the West who sought Hollywood-type entertainment in the clubs (Al Zayer 2004). This style is likely to be performed in restaurants and cabarets all over the world (Shira 2014). Standard costumes consist of bras decorated with lace, beads, or sequins, brightly colored and flowing skirts or harem pants, and coordinating hip scarves or belts to accentuate hip movements (see Figure 1.1). The midriff may or may not be covered. Many American female cabaret dancers display long hair (some dancers with short hair wear wigs or hair extensions). This style of dance is performed solo or in groups and consists of movements that originate from a variety of Middle

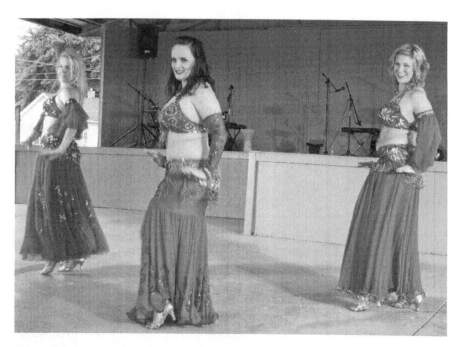

Figure 1.1 American cabaret dance

Eastern and North African countries, such as Egypt, Greece, Turkey, and Lebanon. Solo dances are frequently improvised, while group dances are often choreographed (Al Zayer 2004; Dox 2006; Shay and Sellers-Young 2005).

The cabaret style of belly dance varies slightly by country. For example, the Egyptian style of belly dance, also referred to as Egyptian Oriental, tends to be executed on the balls of the dancer's feet and performed to traditional or modern Egyptian music. Dancers of this style rarely execute floor work, and dancers rarely play zills, or finger cymbals (Farhana 2007). The movements tend to be more isolated, smaller, and controlled compared to other styles of belly dance. Morocco is a pioneer of the Egyptian style of belly dance (Shira 2014). In contrast, the Turkish style is characterized by many turns and hops with backbends and floor work. It is more common for the Turkish style dancer to play zills while performing (Farhana 2007).

Folkloric belly dance is based on traditional dances performed by and for the people in Middle Eastern countries and surrounding areas. These dances generally mimic activities of daily life (Farhana 2007). There are several different types of folkloric dances. One of the most popular is raqs al assaya, also known as an Egyptian cane or staff dance. This dance evolved from men's Egyptian martial arts and a dance known as Tahtib that showcases combat and the handling of weaponry. The cane or staff represents a standard prop used for ordinary and daily tasks, such as walking, plowing, and herding animals. Part of the dance may incorporate balancing the stick on one's head which imitates the people of Egypt balancing items on their head on a daily basis, such as jugs of water or trays of food (El Masri 2010; Jahal 2001).

Another type of folk dance is one based on the Fellahin, the farmers of Egypt. These dances incorporate movements that illustrate the daily activities of farmers, such as gathering food and collecting water (Jahal 2001). Folkloric dances are performed by soloists or groups and can be choreographed or improvised. Folkloric costumes usually cover more of the body and are not as flashy as cabaret costumes (see Figure 1.2).

The tribal and American Tribal Style (proper name of a formal and codified dance) forms of belly dance are rooted in North Africa and dances of the Arabian Peninsula. Jamila Salimpour created the tribal style in San Francisco, California during the 1960s (J. Salimpour 2009). In the 1970s, one of Jamila's students, Masha Archer formed her own group, San Francisco Classic Dance Troupe. Masha sought to distance her dance from the nightclub setting, both in America and the Middle East. Describing her dance as primarily an American style based on Middle Eastern and African roots, Masha altered steps, removed floor work, and performed at events that did not always cater to Middle Eastern culture, such as book fairs and parades. Furthermore, she introduced a chorus of supporting dancers to further distinguish her dance from the lone dancer performing in a nightclub (Archer 2013). As a student of Masha's, Carolena

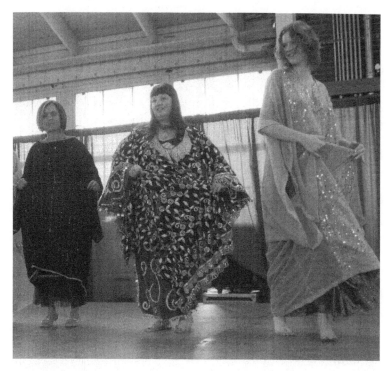

Figure 1.2 Folkloric dance

Nericcio is credited with codifying and registering the American Tribal Style of belly dance around the mid–1980s (Rees-Denis 2008). This dance style is called American Tribal Style because it was organized in the United States, but dancers all over the world participate in this style. For instance, Shades of Araby is one group performing and teaching American Tribal Style currently located in Toronto.

American Tribal Style movements are simple and repetitive to allow for a follow-the-leader routine (Zenuba 2000). This style of belly dance was originally not meant to be performed solo. As its name suggests, dancers form a tribe in which they are constantly communicating with each other during a dance by watching each other for cues, such as eye signals, head turns, and arm movements, to instruct their followers which direction to move in or what step to perform. The tribe typically consists of dancers within the same troupe who are associated with the same studio, perhaps taking classes with the same teacher (Kenny 2007).

Similar to some Afro-Cuban dance that has an element of improvisation (Hagedorn 2001), American Tribal Style is almost never choreographed, although sets of movements may be pre-arranged and rehearsed (Farhana 2007). Rather, American Tribal Style consists of a vocabulary of movements and cues that provide a recognizable structure from which to choose different steps. Far

9

from being completely made up on the spot, dancers have a set of moves from which to spontaneously choose and standardized cues to incorporate to let their fellow dancers know what moves should be executed next. More specifically, American Tribal Style has a vocabulary designated for slow music and a different repertoire of movements for fast songs. Dancers draw from their toolkit of moves based on the tempo of the song to which they are dancing. In most cases, it is expected that the vocabulary for one type of music will not be used for another. During an American Tribal Style act, dancers follow the leader and watch or listen for physical or verbal cues to change steps. Frequently, a dance set will involve more than one leader. At some point during the dance, the leader will join the rest of the group, and another dancer from the group becomes the new leader (Rees-Denis 2008). The dance requires teamwork and cooperation for the dance to be properly executed (Nericcio 2004; Zenuba 2000).

Although the official rhetoric and descriptions of American Tribal Style (ATS) dance emphasize its improvisational nature, formal ATS performances may be less improvisational than social dancing or practicing. Rather, some ATS groups may practice specific sets of moves to particular places in music. They may pre-arrange formations, decide ahead of time who will lead formations and when, and who will provide backup dancing in a chorus behind the main group of dancers.

Whereas cabaret styles of belly dance feature sequins and sparkles on costumes, ATS costumes use natural fabrics, tassel belts, and antique jewelry (Kenny 2007; Zenuba 2000). Costumes tend to include pantaloons (large poofy pants) or harem pants worn underneath full skirts (some made with twenty-five yards of fabric) and choli tops that cover the chest, shoulders, and forearms (Zenuba 2000). Bellies may or may not be covered. The dancers' bodies also become part of the costume with the use of piercings, tattoos, and facial markings (Farhana 2007; Shay and Sellers-Young 2005). ATS dancers also tend to use face adornments, such as bindis (forehead decorations also worn by Hindu women and children) and stick-on jewels, as part of their makeup (Jorgensen 2006; Rees-Denis 2008). Rather than more "flashy" accessories that one may see with cabaret styles of dance, the jewelry tends to showcase charms, coins, and natural materials, such as shells, beads, bone, and pearl (Kenny 2007). Finally, ATS dancers wear their hair pinned up with decorations, such as flowers, or wear short hair that is off the shoulders, which functions to allow dancers' eyes to be visible for movement cues (see Figure 1.3).

Fusion combines one or more styles of belly dance with each other and other dance forms. For example, tribal fusion combines elements of tribal costume and movements with other styles of belly dance and other dances, such as ballet, Bollywood, hip-hop, African, Celtic, vaudeville, or Flamenco. Rachel Brice is at the forefront of tribal fusion dance (Farhana 2007, Rees-Denis 2008).

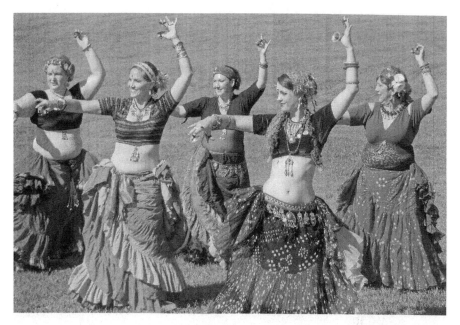

Figure 1.3 American Tribal Style

Photo credit: Scott A. Desmond

Dark fusion is one specific fusion style of belly dance (see Figure 1.4). This style combines elements of belly dance with Goth culture. Performances tend to be highly dramatic, theatrical, and are an outlet for dancers to express the "darker" sides of themselves (Schmidt 2009). Pioneers of this style of dance include Tempest and Ariellah. Fusion dancers may perform to traditional Middle Eastern or more contemporary international and American music (Farhana 2007).

A brief history of belly dance in the West: the lure of the East

Partly based on depictions of the Orient in art and literature, Westerners began creating fantastical images of the Middle East and surrounding areas. Edward Said (1978) refers to this process of eroticizing the Middle East as "Orientalism." In the minds of many Westerners, the Orient symbolized beauty, pleasure, and desire. Images of enticing, sensual, and mysterious women permeated public perceptions. For example, Western ideas of a harem consisted of lavish semi-dressed or nude women dancing for and entertaining men. Despite its longstanding presence in the Middle East and North Africa, and Westerners encountering the dance through their travels to these countries, belly dance did not have a significant presence in the West until the late 1800s.

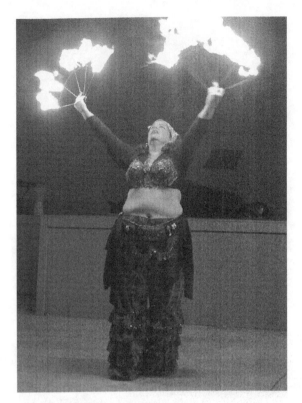

Figure 1.4 Dark fusion belly dance combined with poi

Belly dance on Cairo Street

In the late nineteenth century, a series of fairs and world exhibitions were held in the United States, France, and Great Britain that displayed various dancers from Middle Eastern and surrounding countries that gave rise to interest in "exotic" dance forms (Shay 2008). During his visit to the 1889 Paris Exposition Universelle, Sol Bloom, a relatively young and wealthy businessman, was intrigued by women he saw dancing in an Algerian village. Sol arranged to bring these dancers to the United States to perform as part of the 1893 World's Fair in Chicago (Carlton 1994).

The Midway Plaisance was a subdivision of the Chicago World's Fair that displayed working villages modeled after those in their native countries, such as Algeria, Turkey, and Egypt. Cairo Street was a particularly noteworthy and popular area. This area featured "dancing girls" performing dances from their homelands which emphasized the core of the body (Al Zayer 2004; Carlton 1994). The Midway Plaisance, and the dancers, are said to have been the fair's most popular attraction. It was one of the only areas to draw large crowds on Sunday when it was controversial for the fair to even be open (Carlton 1994).

Although the dancers were very popular, they also sparked much controversy (Shay and Sellers-Young 2005). During this Victorian Age, women's bodies were tightly constrained with corsets and heavily clothed. Exposing a female ankle was considered risqué (Al Zayer 2004). The dancers' unrestrained rotations and gyrations of the pelvis, hips, and stomach deviated from bodily movements deemed acceptable at the time and were considered morally offensive (Shay and Sellers-Young 2005). Because their movements were disturbing to some onlookers, officials, such as Anthony Comstock (for whom the 1873 anti-obscenity Comstock Act is named), attempted to shut down the performances, enticing more people to see the shows (for more detail, see Carlton 1994). After the fair, venues continued offering belly dance performances because they drew large crowds. Erotic displays attracted even greater audiences, so some belly dance acts became more sexualized. Burlesque houses adopted the dance, and belly dance became linked to burlesque, erotic dance, and sex work (Carlton 1994; Sellers-Young 1992; Shira 2014).

Beyond Cairo Street

The increasing popularity of movies, stage productions, and music during the first half of the twentieth century portraying Westernized images of the East heightened Americans' awareness of belly dance (Carlton 1994; Sellers-Young 1992; Shira 2014). Ballets, such as Scheherazade (Russian) and the Nutcracker, and Salome (a stage production based on the biblical story of John the Baptist), include Arabian themes and Oriental images (Carlton 1994; Shay and Sellers-Young 2005). Although it could be argued that these productions catered to "Orientalist" visions, the performances showcased the Orient and belly dance within "classy" settings outside of burlesque houses that some people considered less respectable.

Along with the increase in film and stage productions, the Immigration and Nationality Act of 1965 loosened bans on immigration from several areas of the world. As a result, greater numbers of Arabs, Jews, and Muslims from North Africa and the Middle East immigrated to America (Le 2009). In some parts of the United States, an upsurge of restaurants and clubs specializing in Middle Eastern food provided a meeting place for Middle Eastern and North African immigrants from countries including Egypt, Iraq, Turkey, and Lebanon (Sellers-Young 2009; Shay and Sellers-Young 2005). These clubs and restaurants showcased various musicians and dancers performing professional Middle Eastern dance (Shay 2008).

At the same time that these clubs opened, belly dance also became linked to the feminist movement (Sellers-Young 1992; Shay and Sellers-Young 2005). Among other goals, the women's movement of the 1960s and 1970s encouraged women to adopt a more liberated approach toward physical expression and their own sexual desires (Shay and Sellers-Young 2005). With its focus on engaging the stomach, hips, shoulders, and chest, belly dance was viewed as one way to meet this call for female expression (Dox 2006; Sellers-Young 1992). The women's movement advocated that feminine bodies should be free and expressive rather than hidden or confined, which sharply contrasts with early twentieth-century customs (Shay 2008). Some female dancers considered the dance an empowering path for women to become more aware of their bodies, experience sexual subjectivity, and gain some control over the male gaze (Dox 2006; Sellers-Young 1992; Shay 2008). Shay (2008) argues that the construction of belly dance as a way to experience this newfound freedom contributed to the rise of its popularity. During this time, thousands of middle-class, primarily white, American women sought to learn new dance forms (Shay 2008). By the 1980s, over one million women had signed up for belly dance classes all over the United States (Sellers-Young 1992).

Along with feminism and the sexual revolution, Shay (2008) claims that women sought to create new and "exotic" identities and constructed belly dance as a pathway to do just that. By "exotic," Shay means exciting, beautiful, and unknown. Because dance is an embodied form of cultural production involving costumes, music, alternative names, and accessories, belly dance stage performances and social dancing work toward this end (Shay 2008). Shay (2008) argues that some Americans sought alternative identities because people who grew up in the 1940s through the 1970s rarely saw or interacted with people who did not look like them due to a social climate saturated with racism, discrimination, and segregation. In response to these prevailing social conditions, many Americans looked for opportunities to embrace and learn about cultural diversity. Furthermore, some Americans felt like they did not have their own cultural roots. Being a "white" American was perceived by many as having a non-distinct identity that lacked uniqueness and an intriguing cultural heritage. Dance gave people a break from racism and segregation, while providing tools to construct a more culturally interesting identity. Participating in "exotic" dance forms, such as belly dance, and borrowing elements from other cultures, provided some depth and meaning to participants' lives. They interpreted these dances as real, authentic, historical, and part of a simple past filled with deep values (for an extensive discussion of historical trends during the twentieth century that gave rise to American interest in belly dance and other "exotic" dance forms, see Shay 2008).

All of these events of early Orientalist film and stage portrayals, the feminist movement and sexual revolution, and borrowing from other cultures to construct an alternative "exotic" identity influence people's experience with belly dance today, which shape the focus of this book. Therefore, like many other forms of dance, such as ballroom (Marion 2008), Afro-Cuban Santeria (Hagedorn 2001), and ballet (Wulff 1998), belly dance is more than just a physical enterprise. There is a social and cultural context that surrounds all dance genres.

A belly dance (sub)culture

Similar to ballroom dance (Marion 2008) and tango (Savigliano 1998), belly dance is a subculture that is distinguished from many participants' ordinary lives. "It's kind of like the underworld . . . This community is a world of its own," Laurel replies when I ask her about the benefits she receives from belly dance that she does not get in other contexts. Although people may see belly dance at shows, festivals, or on television, to an outsider, belly dance may appear mysterious. Because she views the social world of belly dance as unique and "something that [most] people just don't do," Laurel thinks "it's wonderful."

Strauss (1978) brought the concept of social worlds to the forefront of academic inquiry at a level of analysis between individuals and social structures. Unruh (1980:277) defines a social world as a collection of "actors, organizations, events, and practices which have coalesced into spheres of interest and involvement for participants. It is likely that a powerful centralized authority structure does not exist." Social worlds consist of common knowledge, norms, values, shared space, relationships, and communities. Belly dance is a national community with networks of classes, workshops, instructors who travel all over the world, magazines, newsletters, a slew of internet sites, and regional and national conventions (Shay 2008). These social worlds are arenas in which people participate and communicate and around which people organize social life (Clarke and Friese 2007; Strauss 1978).

Social worlds consist of multiple groups and interlocking networks that each have their own culture. These individual and small groups have their own cultures that are described as "idiocultures" (Fine 2012a). A group's "idioculture" consists of the "shared beliefs, ideas, knowledge, and behaviors" that serve as a "frame of reference and basis of interaction for group members" (Fine 1987:125). These cultures contain a wide range of clothing styles, nicknames, jokes, slang terminology, rules of conduct, and music (Fine 1987). As group members interact with each other and communicate with members of other groups, broader cultural traditions develop. These customs become expectations that guide the interactions and behaviors of their members (Strauss 1964). In other words, we define ourselves by the use of shared symbols within the cultures in which we participate. By belonging to different groups, individuals construct alternative identities as part of their sense of self (Fine 2012b).

Small group cultures within belly dance occur in different forms. They may be the people who make up a weekly classes or workshop attendees. Classes may consist of five to twenty students, and thirty to one hundred people may attend a single workshop. A group may also consist of a collectivity of dancers who often practice and perform with one another – a troupe. Belly dance troupes also have a leader who is typically the primary instructor of classes and the organizer/founder of troupes associated with his/her classes. Troupe members take cues from the leader regarding appropriate behavior, dance, and costuming. Erica, a seasoned dancer and former instructor remarks, "It's the instructor [troupe leader] who sets the tone for the group."

There are various avenues through which ideas are communicated across different groups (Fine 2002). First, some people may belong to multiple groups; thereby cultural traditions within one collectivity may spread to others. For instance, some belly dancers simultaneously take classes with several instructors. Alternatively, some dancers offer instruction to one class and receive instruction from another teacher. Furthermore, dancers may attend or perform at each other's haflas (belly dance party typically consisting of formal performances and some open dancing) and events. A hafla taking place in one city may host performers from surrounding areas. Therefore, even though regular participation in belly dance usually occurs in small groups, these collectivities are often well connected and people easily move between them.

Along with maintaining connections to multiple groups, Fine (2002) suggests that communication across groups occurs through weak ties. Many dance forms, such as ballroom (Marion 2008), have organizations dedicated to advancing the art and bringing together dancers from different groups. In addition to regular involvement in small groups, belly dancers are sometimes loosely connected to one another through their affiliations with local and national organizations. Examples of these organizations include the Indiana Association of Middle Eastern Teachers and Dancers, North Texas Middle Eastern Dance Association, and the San Diego Area Middle Eastern Dance Association. Belly dance organizations exist to educate the public about the activity, and some organizations sponsor dance-related workshops and performances to advance the teaching and performance of the dance form. These organizations dictate etiquette and rules and provide a framework and structure for dancers who participate in these various organizations' events. For instance, leaders of at least one belly dance organization require performers at their events to cover their stomachs either with colored belly covers, leotards, shirts, or the like. One purpose of this guideline is to preserve Middle Eastern and North African culture in which women did and do not typically belly dance with their stomachs exposed.

In addition, there are numerous digital and print magazines devoted to the lives and experiences of belly dancers. Two popular online magazines are *The*

Gilded Serpent and *Zaghareet*. Both of these resources feature articles on various aspects of belly dance, including individual dancers, troupes, music, musicians, history, travel, and styles of dance. Also, several websites and Internet groups devoted to belly dance have emerged. There are currently over five hundred belly dance groups on Facebook alone.

Along with magazines and Internet resources, dancers network with each other at workshops and festivals. A workshop may draw dancers from neighboring states and national events may attract dancers from several parts of the country. For instance, Yaa Halla Y'all is an annual event that takes place in Texas. Over multiple days, Yaa Halla Y'all offers workshops with instructors from all around the country. In the evenings, workshop instructors and dancers perform a variety of belly dance styles. Similarly, Rakkasah hosts four Middle Eastern dance festivals throughout the year. Rakkasah West is considered to be the largest belly dance festival in the world. The festivals offer workshops with internationally known dancers and music teachers. Multiple stages feature a variety of bands. Tribal Revolution is an annual multi-day tribal fusion event in Chicago that draws belly dancers from all over the United States. A wide range of classes are offered and various dancers are showcased in performances. Vendors sell a variety of belly dance related costumes and accessories. Although attendees do not see each other on a daily basis, they meet one another for a short period of time and form ties at these festivals.

There are several norms and values that operate within belly dance. Some norms are particularly relevant during belly dance performances. A single show typically features multiple performers. A standard rule of belly dance etiquette is for performers to wear cover-ups, such as a long jacket, veil, or shirt, over their costumes until it is time to perform to make the biggest impact possible when their costumes are unveiled. In addition, because belly dance costumes are frequently judged as beautiful, some believe that revealing one's costume during someone else's act detracts attention away from the performer. Likewise, when a belly dancer takes the stage, other performers are expected to watch the act rather than leave or busy themselves with other activities, which may be considered rude. If people are moving around near the stage, the audience may be distracted and turn their attention away from the performer. For instance, during a performance at one hafla I attended, a few dancers who had yet to perform sat near the front of the audience. They searched for costume pieces and tried to locate their music to prepare for their act. Their director reminded them that they needed to remain still if they wanted to sit up front or they should move toward the back of the room if they needed to finish getting ready for their performance.

Audiences are considered active participants in some dance shows, such as ballroom showcases (Marion 2008). Likewise, belly dance audiences are not removed from performances. Dancers frequently interact with the onlookers and appreciate feedback, such as clapping and supportive verbal cues during a performance. To set the tone for audience participation during a belly dance show, emcees talk with audiences about the importance of applause and appropriate noises to make during performances in the hopes of increasing audience involvement during the show. For instance, emcees frequently teach audience members how to zaghareet. Zaghareet is an ululation in which someone quickly repeats "La, La, La" using a high-pitched voice. It was used in the context of war as a battle cry and to welcome home military troupes. It is also used as an expression of joy in any place people gather, such as festivals and weddings. One is likely to hear a zaghareet at belly dance performances as a sign of enjoying the act and to direct audiences' attention toward a performer.

Along with various norms, idiocultures contain a special language or jargon to identify objects that are important to the group, and belly dance is no exception. It is important to note that because there are many belly dance groups, performers, and instructors, language and terminology can vary across people and places. As I mentioned earlier, a hafla generally refers to a gathering or party that may include dancers, musicians, and vendors of belly dance paraphernalia. Haflas may consist of formal dance performances and informal open dancing available to anyone in attendance. Music accompanying performances may be recorded or performed live. Zills, also known as "sills" or "sagat" in some areas of the world, are finger cymbals used as musical instruments to accompany some people while they belly dance. Zills may be played by performers, musicians, or audience members.

Setting the stage

Chapter 2 begins our journey into how participants use cultural resources within belly dance to create a sense of self and build social relationships. In this chapter I analyze gender performance and explore how both men and women construct masculinities and femininities within belly dance. Female dancers enact different versions of femininity. Some draw symbolic lines around "dainty" and "powerful" feminine beauty through the use of costumes and movements. Like many women, male dancers utilize several strategies to "do" masculinity. How these men emphasize traditional notions of masculinity and the extent to which those performances are successful hinge on the dance community in which they participate.

In Chapter 3, I examine agreed upon and contested messages surrounding the body and how these ideals are influenced by larger Western cultural standards. I pay particular attention to the preponderance of body-positive messages inside belly dance circles and how many aspects of belly dance support body acceptance. At the same time, I consider how these body-positive values change once dancers leave their local communities and perform for a general audience. I analyze various mechanisms dancers use to both alter and cover their bodies in response to these larger cultural expectations. Furthermore, I explore the highly contested arena of sexuality and consider how internal debates are situated in cultural ambivalence about (female) sexuality. Finally, I note how men's bodily experiences in belly dance greatly contrast with that of female dancers, particularly noting the pervasive lack of sexualizing belly dance among male dancers.

That belly dance is a gendered bodily endeavor has important implications for the relationships that are created inside this social world. As a female-dominated leisure space, belly dance is first and foremost a highly gendered (feminized) location for women to form bonds with one another when they may not have the opportunity in their professions or other social outlets. Chapter 4 examines how participants do friendship within belly dance and characteristics of the dance that support the building of these relationships. I consider how the relatively flat hierarchical structure, costumes, and performance opportunities help facilitate positive interactions between dancers. I highlight how interlocking networks and overlapping memberships across belly dance groups strengthen relationships that defy geographic boundaries.

In Chapter 5, I examine how male and female dancers define belly dance in ways that support or prohibit the dance from becoming spiritually meaningful. How participants think of belly dance as spiritual is based on their various experiences within the dance, dancing in different contexts, performing with certain people, moving to particular music, and how they conceptualize both belly dance and spirituality. For dancers who infuse the activity with spiritual meaning, specific movements and music can become meditative or ritualistic in ways that allow dancers to enter "flow." In other words, people become so intensely involved in an activity that they forget about everything else around them. They lose track of time and their surroundings because they are completely absorbed in the activity. Illustrating the constructed nature of spirituality, I also consider how spirituality is inhibited, focusing on how some people define the dance and spirituality as incompatible, while some dancers simply do not see themselves as spiritual people. Furthermore, people who "work" too much at belly dance, such as some teachers and novice students, are less likely to infuse the activity with spiritual meaning. Along these same lines, I consider how time can either help or hinder dancers associating spirituality with belly dance.

Belly dance is a site for identity construction and offers a variety of tools with which dancers can experiment. The extent to which people acknowledge and abide by the norms of the larger belly dance community and their specific group's idioculture has implications for identity work. In Chapter 6, I explore expectations associated with the role of belly dancer. The varying

degrees to which people adhere to and internalize these norms have consequences for how dancers construct and confer a belly dance label. I pay special attention to various role-making and role-taking strategies dancers use to
adopt (or not) stage names as one particular marker of identity within some
dance communities.

In Chapters 7 and 8, I explore various challenges participants encounter as
belly dancers. A paucity of scholarly attention is paid to the costs that people
manage by participating in leisure communities, and these issues are almost
never explored in adult, female-dominated leisure subcultures. In Chapter 7,
I examine the challenges inside the world of belly dance, such as issues of legitimacy, power, and status hierarchies, along with debates that focus on authenticity. These issues shed light on competition for performance opportunities and
cattiness, which contaminate women's friendships. Because they are typically
sought out for different performances, male dancers are practically immune to
the competitive issues that plague relationships between female dancers.

As a subculture that frequently interacts with and is shared with the
larger culture, belly dancers routinely manage interactions with outsiders. In
Chapter 8, I examine how dancers confront perceptions that belly dance is
inappropriately and overtly sexual. Women manage perceptions that they are
hyper sexual, available for a heterosexual man's pleasure, and behave like erotic
dancers. On the other hand, men manage attacks on their masculinity and perceptions they are gay. Although they navigate somewhat different public ideas,
both male and female dancers engage in numerous management strategies to
mitigate stigma attached to belly dance.

Chapter 9 concludes the book. As a leisure subculture, I reiterate the various benefits and challenges of participating in the social world of belly dance.
I revisit how belly dance is primarily a form of leisure that allows dancers to
play with gender, identity construction, friendships, and spirituality that are
somewhat different from their lives outside of belly dance. I consider how the
unique characteristics of belly dance, as a dance form rooted in another culture in which the participants constantly interact with the general public, have
important implications for how female and male participants construct their
identities, perform gender, navigate friendships, create spiritual experiences,
and manage (often ill-perceived) public attitudes.

Although this book is about American belly dance, it is about far more
than dancing. Rather, it focuses on the people who are involved in this dance
and the culture(s) that surround it. Dance forms cannot execute themselves.
They are brought alive by people (Marion 2008). Because dance is intentional,
deliberate, and requires work, it reflects and shapes larger cultural and social
norms (Marion 2008). In turn, these norms influence and are influenced by
the people who participate in dance. I invite you into the world of American
belly dance.

Chapter 2

Performing gender

While working toward my Master's degree at Purdue University, I write a thesis guided by a committee of all but one men, and my advisor is male. As a graduate assistant, I work with only male professors. Once I finish my M.A., I begin my Ph.D. course work and plan a dissertation with a four-person committee consisting of all men. Furthermore, I help manage a survey research lab with a male boss and almost all male co-workers. I feel overwhelmed interacting with so many men in my professional life. I'm ready to play with femininity and share some space with women. In this chapter, I explore how many women use belly dance to construct femininities, while, to varying degrees, male dancers "do" masculinity.

Doing gender refers to how we perform masculine and feminine traits through bodily gestures and movement (Connell 2002; Goffman 1959; Stets and Burke 2009; West and Zimmerman 1987). We do or construct gender partly based on the messages we receive about how we are supposed to look and act for the gender with which we identify (Clarke 2011; Howard 2000). We present ourselves as masculine or feminine within the frameworks that are provided by cultural scripts (Butler 1988, 1990; Connell 2002). Boys are taught from an early age to behave in socially approved masculine ways, while girls are expected to act in accordance with cultural ideas of femininity (Schrock and Schwalbe 2009). Some people resist these binary categories of male and female, preferring different gendered labels or no gender identifier. However, belly dance is a site in which dancers express fairly traditional dichotomous notions of masculinity and femininity.

As an embodied pursuit, dance is a vehicle through which we negotiate gender and its performance (Burt 2009). How dancers move and present their bodies confirms or challenges notions of masculinity and femininity (Fisher and Shay 2009; Marion 2008). How, where, when, how long, and why people dance, who dances, and how they are dressed communicate quite a bit about gender (Marion 2008).

"I feel like I live in a man's world"

Because most belly dancers in the United States are women (Sellers-Young 1992),[1] dance classes, workshops, and rehearsals provide settings in which women are relatively free from a male gaze. Participating in belly dance gives some women a break from other aspects of life that are saturated with men, while offering them tools to express femininity. Workplaces are sites for gender divisions and can take on qualities of femininity or masculinity (Connell 2002). Several women in this study have careers in fields that are typically dominated by men, such as the natural sciences, management and finance, medicine, and technology, and/or they work with primarily male co-workers.

In her mid-twenties, Angelica is in graduate school working toward a music degree. Belly dance is therapeutic for Angelica because, "I just get bogged down. I feel like I live in a man's world," she says. "It's hard not to feel at the end of the day that I've made a lot of concessions on the things I think and the things I feel for what a man wants." Angelica is working on a music project with a male colleague, and they have difficulty reaching a consensus. Although the project was originally Angelica's idea, "I feel myself almost saying 'oh it's Ok. We can do what you want.'" Belly dance helps Angelica "feel empowered and recharged." The dance reminds her "not to fold under this male pressure in society and relationships."

"I always felt a bit out of place," Leah tells me. "I was a girl with the best grades in my class who liked science more than liberal arts." She claims that she has "always been strange" as a woman who has a Ph.D. in mathematics. Although she generally feels isolated in her profession – "there is a little bit of everything [in her belly dance classes] except there tends to be a common science theme" – Leah's observations mirror my initial impressions of my first dance class. "[Her getting involved in belly dance] might have been triggered by the fact there were no women around and, I felt the need to do more feminine [activities]," she explains. Partly because she works in a male-dominated field with primarily men, Leah wanted to participate in a feminine activity that would facilitate her interacting with other women.

"What has kept you in belly dance all this time?" I ask Brooke who has been involved in belly dance for over thirty years. "I got in touch with my femininity by doing this dance," she responds. Brooke calls herself "a farm girl that was just kind of a little hippie chick." Now in her fifties, she explains that belly dance "really got me in touch with this feminine side, because I was always a tomboy growing up." Over time, she began to "adore" the "beauty and glamour" that she found in belly dance. "It's so much fun to dress up and to have an alter ego!" Although Brooke does not work in a masculine dominated setting, as a "farm girl," she did not have many opportunities to express femininity. Dancers like Angelica, Leah, and Brooke enjoy belly dance partly because they feel validated and "empowered" as women. They feel that as women in male-dominated settings, they do not have as strong a voice, and feel isolated or less respected. Belly dance helps them affirm their strength and value as women and provides tools to play with femininity that aren't typically available to them in their everyday lives. At the core of these resources lies the very distinct clothing worn by belly dancers. The beauty and glamor Brooke refers to in belly dance hints at the role costumes play in how female dancers construct femininity.

"I almost always wear some pink when I perform"

In his ethnography of competitive ballroom dance, Jonathan Marion (2008), refers to ballroom as a "spectacle" in that dancers' costumes are designed to showcase their bodies and enhance their movements for the purpose of being viewed. The costumes and movements communicate "maleness" and "femaleness." Much like standard attire for swimmers (Scott 2009), belly dance costumes cover traditionally sexualized body parts, while also enhancing them. Decorated bras, a core component of a typical female belly dance costume, cover and simultaneously enhance the breasts. Furthermore, large hip scarves draw attention to and accentuate hip movements.

Clothing, in general, communicates to both the wearer and onlookers. It can influence a person's attitude and behavior, i.e. a woman may feel better about herself when she wears an outfit that she feels highlights her positive features while downplaying less appealing physical assets. In this sense, clothing becomes a "second skin" (Goffman 1974) in that what we wear penetrates us and becomes a little of who we are. At the same time, clothing choices influence how other people respond to us, e.g. treating us with greater respect if they judge us as professional. Some female belly dancers feel more attractive when they are dressed in belly dance costumes and audiences compliment them on their appearance. Although there is a debate in the academic literature regarding whether beauty-work is creative, empowering, and enjoyable (Beausoleil 1994; Weitz 2001) or whether it is repressive and keeps women insecure (Bordo 2003; Hesse-Biber 2006), Clarke (2011) argues that the pleasure women receive from beauty practices is rooted in their ability to achieve a culturally accepted appearance. Dress, makeup, and gestures mark the production of femaleness and womanhood in our culture (Beausoleil 1994). Costumes are one of the most common tools that female dancers use to help them feel more feminine. Dancers judge long skirts, flowers, bright colors, sequins, and sparkles as expressions of womanhood. "It emphasizes femininity, and I like that," Shelby says. "Part of it probably is because my job is such a man-oriented job, and I don't get to dress pretty, and my hair is forever braided . . . I wear work clothes, jeans, and steel toed boots that are covered in gunk. This is a way that I can definitely be womanly." Like several dancers, Shelby suggests that belly dance affords her the opportunity to wear stereotypical feminine clothing that she does not generally wear in her working life.

When Peg was younger, she "hated being a girlie girl." She didn't like the color pink or clothing marketed toward little girls. However, she was involved in theater and enjoyed dressing up for her various performances. "You mean I can wear all of this weird stuff outside of the theater?" Peg says about finding belly dance. "I was allowed to be a girlie girl, I was allowed to sit there and play with my makeup for an hour because it was for a performance. I was allowed to buy these outrageous colors that clash. I was allowed to wear glitter. I was allowed to wear sequins, and it was OK," Peg continues. Peg attended Catholic school as a child and wearing bright colors and shiny fabric wasn't acceptable. "You weren't allowed to stand out. You weren't allowed to do anything out of the norm," Peg remembers. Dressing in belly dance costumes provides an opportunity for dancers like Peg to feel more feminine.

Alexandra entered the world of belly dance while she was working on a Ph.D. in history. Strained interactions with her advisor helped her realize she wanted to explore her creativity and femininity. As a graduate student instructor, Alexandra had difficulty maintaining authority in her classroom. She talked with her advisor about her concerns, and she interpreted her advisor's response as wanting her to "dress in a more boring, dowdy, less feminine fashion." Alexandra's advisor did not want her to wear skirts or makeup and told her to stop wearing bangs along with her long hair. "I think I was looking for something more feminine because at work I was encouraged not to be feminine . . . [Her advisor] thought that the feminine [attire] was undermining my authority in the classroom," she tells me. "I don't know that I was consciously aware that I wanted something feminine and girly and pink and frilly in my life, but belly dance is an opportunity to be girly," she explains. In this way, Alexandra used much of the standard costumes and norms for hair and makeup within belly dance to express her femininity which she felt she could not do in her professional life. "I don't know why belly dance became the symbolic rebellion," Alexandra begins. She continues:

> I almost always wear my hair down when I belly dance, and toss it around. Maybe that is why I like the cabaret and nightclub style, because [her advisor] thought that dressing in an overly feminine manner, wearing pink or pastels, or ruffles, or lace, or – heaven forbid – sparkles, was undermining any authority I would have in the classroom. So of course, my first belly dance costume was pink and sparkly. In fact, I almost always wear some pink when I perform.

Here Alexandra explains that those wardrobe components that her advisor used to mark (and disapprove of) as feminine are the same tools she uses in belly dance to enhance and express her notion of femininity.

"You've got the graceful movements"

"I started to crave that delicious expression of femininity that belly dance offers," Lydia begins as we sit on the steps outside of the building where she has just finished her weekly dance class. "How is belly dance an expression of femininity?" I ask. Although Lydia recognizes that men are also involved in the dance, "it's moving in a way that accentuates the feminine aspects of my body," she replies.

Similar to Lydia, Laurel has always thought that belly dance is very beautiful. "What do you find so beautiful about it?" I ask her. "I just think it's very feminine and it's very artistic," she replies. "You've got the graceful movements," Laurel continues. She associates ballet movements with grace, and "I can see a lot of ballet movements in [belly dance]," Laurel explains.

Belly dance movements, which Lydia and Laurel define as feminine, can be graceful in several ways. First, proper posture is strongly emphasized across a variety of dance styles. Good posture is typically defined as standing tall, knees slightly bent, shoulders rolled down and back, the head and chest lifted. Second, particular arm movements may be considered graceful. Several instructors guide students to raise and lower their arms by engaging muscles in the upper back, biceps, and triceps rather than leading the movement with the hands, wrists, or forearms. Arm movements originating from the upper arm and back are typically judged more attractive. Finally, executing movements that flow together rather than being jagged with abrupt starts and stops is deemed graceful. If a move looks too mechanical and robotic, it may lack grace. In all of these ways, female dancers attempt to move gracefully, which some associate with femininity.

There are many examples of men potentially being described as "graceful" within the context of sports. However, male dancers typically do not emphasize grace as a part of masculine belly dance. My intention is not to suggest that men cannot be graceful belly dancers, but only that women appear to claim this word as an expression of femininity within belly dance. Men talk about movements emphasizing masculinity in other ways that I will discuss later in this chapter.

Resisting the "dainty"

Some female dancers construct femininity as combining beauty with strength in belly dance. Although empowerment is a word that many female dancers use to talk about their experiences across dance styles, it is not uncommon for tribal, especially American Tribal Style, dancers to construct femininity as a combination of attractiveness and power. It has been argued that the American

Tribal Style of belly dance critiques traditional Western notions of femininity (Kenny 2007). In some ways, it crosses boundaries of masculinity and femininity by showcasing female dancers demonstrating power and strength, while maintaining stereotypical notions of beauty. Hegemonic masculinity postulates that traditional masculinity, such as power and strength, is a goal for both men and women. In this way, both men and women can "safely" strive to embody masculine traits, while men are not encouraged to embrace femininity (Wade and Ferree 2015).

In American Tribal Style, proper posture focuses on lengthening the torso to stand up straight while holding slightly curved arms at chest level or overhead (Kenny 2007). When we hold our bodies in expanded and lifted ways, we fill space, which instills a sense of power. Power is gendered. We typically think of men's physical bodies taking up more space and women holding themselves with more deference (Wade and Ferree 2015). Furthermore, femininity is done partly by smiling sweetly at someone (Wade and Ferree 2015). "I view cabaret as being kind of coy," Cameron tells me. "I like tribal because it seems more down to earth, and that's how I view myself. It seems more earthy without any façade or pretense," she continues. Cameron believes that tribal dancers dance primarily for the enjoyment of dancing, whereas cabaret dancers are more "cute" and "a little flirty," she tells me. "I am just not like that. I wouldn't have been able to pull that off. So this is much more like me."

Like Cameron, Agnes says about American Tribal Style dancing, "It's a very grounded style . . . The posture is different between tribal and cabaret. Your hips are tilted a little more sharply, and your knees are bent a little more. I think about sinking my weight into the ground a little further," she begins. However, when she started learning cabaret, she felt like she was "floating." "Tribal is just very down to earth, very grounded, and I like that," Agnes remarks.

One Saturday, I attend an American Tribal Style workshop that is led by a well-known American Tribal Style dancer. The teacher instructs us to stand tall with our arms firmly lifted at chest height to execute a particular move. She says our body posture and movement should illustrate strength and beauty rather than being dainty. When we converse after the workshop about her instruction, she remarks, "We as ATS dancers hope to promote strength, beauty, and grace with the dance. The way we hold our posture, the way we lead, how we hold our props with confidence and strength," she begins. "What did you mean when you talked about being dainty?" I ask. "We are not really a dainty dance. Nothing wrong with dainty at all, but holding firmly our props with the elbows and chest lifted gives off an amazing look," she explains. Without explicitly saying so, this instructor differentiates American Tribal Style dance from some other forms of belly dance that may be characterized as softer.

Some cabaret dancers also distinguish their dance from tribal in similar ways to how tribal dancers distinguish their dance from cabaret. Tribal is "More earthy, more in touch with what you are doing. In a night club they are more free, and in tribal or folk I think it is more earth and power," Rose tells me. She prefers the freedom and showiness of the cabaret style because she says, "I'm a cheese cake. I like that." Like Cameron, Rose suggests that her preferred style of dance fits her personality.

Regardless of style, many women enjoy dressing in hyperfeminine costumes, fixing their hair, and wearing a lot of makeup and jewelry. At the same time, various types of femininity are presented by different dancers. The version of femininity that is showcased depends on the style of belly dance. Specifically, some dancers suggest cabaret styles project one type of femininity that is lighter, while tribal styles display earthiness and being grounded.

Performing masculinity

Understanding global history and globalization is crucial for studies of masculinity. Western imperialism, colonialism, and global markets have great implications for gender performance and relationships today. Western culture has circulated around the world and influences local ideas and definitions of masculinity. Colonizing people have problematized the masculinity of the people with whom they come in contact, and those colonizing people work to change gender norms (Connell 2005; Kimmel 2005). The male experience in Middle Eastern dance is no exception. In many parts of the Middle East, attitudes toward both male and female dancers were quite ambivalent. On one hand, dancers were popular and celebrated as creative artists. In fact, dancers were highly sought-after for various celebrations, such as weddings and festivals. On the other hand, performers were also often ostracized, labeled as prostitutes, and ridiculed. Both men and women suffered from these negative attitudes, but perhaps men more so since dancing is regarded as an activity more appropriate for women than for men (Fisher and Shay 2009).

Old Middle Eastern dance traditions changed over time in response to colonial disapproval and generally negative attitudes toward dance. Historically, both male and female dancers performed very similar movements and styles (Karayanni 2009; Shay 2009). However, Europeans only enjoyed typical Middle Eastern dance if it was performed by women. Male Middle Eastern dancers performing controlled movements of the torso, pelvis, and chest offended many Westerners who believed that movements of those body parts were reserved solely for women. Therefore, in Egypt, and to varying degrees in Iran and Uzbekistan, hypermasculine styles of the dance were created to appease Westerners and Western elite preferences. These invented male dances emphasized skips, hops, steps that cover large spaces of dance area, and strong hand and arm gestures that appear rigid. Unlike traditional forms of Middle

Eastern dance, again performed by both men and women, these newly con-structed male movements require the torso to remain firm, while reducing shoulder shimmies and pelvic movements. Furthermore, rather than being showcased, male dancers were expected to serve as backdrops for the featured female dancers. They were instructed to play stereotypically masculine roles and assume traditional masculine poses while the women danced around them. Also, their dances often incorporated the use of sticks and swords to mimic martial arts movements (Shay 2009). Because confrontation is symbolically masculine, other behaviors (such as dance) that are deemed less masculine might be forgiven within the context of fighting (Ferguson 2000). Therefore, inserting fighting movements and symbols into dance functions to elevate masculinity within an otherwise feminine context. As a result, when dancers draw on masculinized notions of belly dance, they are generally invoking these post-colonial Western constructs. In this section, I examine how men perform masculinity within the female-dominated setting of belly dance.

Similar to ballet and jazz (Fisher 2009; Mennesson 2009), even when men are present in classes, belly dance instruction is typically geared toward women. In our everyday culture, "guys" is the default pronoun to refer to a group of people regardless of the gender makeup (I frequently catch myself referring to the mixed-gender student collectivity in my sociology of gender class as "guys"). Being sensitive to the gender makeup in belly dance classes, some instructors refer to the group as "ladies." Indicative of the social expectation for the collective to be referred to as "guys," when I ask Henry what it's like to navigate a world dominated by women, he replies, "In our society, it's male dominated, but in belly dance its female dominated. It's an interesting per-spective to be a minority in a minority." "Do you feel like a minority?" I ask. "Occasionally when I'm at workshops someone will say 'Ok ladies,' and I'm comfortable enough in who I am if someone uses the collective word ladies and I'm the only guy, it's not an offense," Henry replies. Although Henry claims that outside of the context of a dance class, a man might take offense at being included in a group of ladies. However, women being included in a group of "guys" is culturally less problematic. In other words, "guys" is more universal and acceptable across genders, while "ladies" is specifically gendered and appropriate mostly for women.

"I'm not gay"

For his work on masculinity, Kimmel (2008) asked men how they know whether a guy is gay. The responses pointed to stereotypically effeminate behaviors, such as his dress and if he is interested in art or music. Liking art and music automatically puts men at a social disadvantage because some people

28

will question their sexual orientation, and thus their manhood. Brooke tells me about a male dancer who walked into her class and immediately announced, "I'm not gay." Regardless of this student's sexuality, it is noteworthy that he felt it necessary to let everyone know that he isn't attracted to members of his own sex. He responds to cultural assumptions that men who participate in belly dance are probably gay. His comments publicly reaffirm his heterosexuality thereby protecting at least one aspect of his masculinity.

"This even falls back on my sexuality, sometimes I feel more aggressive," Denny tells me. "I can grow out my facial hair and stomp around with sticks on stage and be very grrrr. [I can be] very masculine or very machismo and show that masculine side of me. That's one of the big things that I like about it." Denny's comments draw on several aspects of hegemonic masculinity. Hegemonic masculinity refers to an idealized man who embodies the most desirable traits of manhood, such as being strong, successful, powerful, and sexually active (Connell 1987). For a man to enjoy the privileges of being a man, he must act in ways to credibly establish himself as a man, such as demon-strating violence, aggression, and sexual prowess (Schrock and Schwalbe 2009). Masculinity is reinforced through warrior images and sports that emphasize competition, dominance, and the ability to control others or at least avoid being controlled (Schrock and Schwalbe 2009). Although male belly dancers do not typically emphasize sexuality in their dance, as I will discuss in the next chapter, Denny draws on traditional notions of hegemonic masculinity that include a sexual appetite to partly construct his ideas about manhood.

"It's a very masculine style"

Some male dancers argue that various styles of belly dance are more conducive to portraying masculinity. Denny claims that "there are different styles that may look better for a male dancer." He believes that the tribal style involves a lot of aggres-sion. He thinks men can perform it better because, "visually sometimes it is more appealing...That's one of the important things about having male belly dancers," he explains. About the tribal style of dance, Denny remarks, "to me, it's a very mas-culine style. I like that a lot ... it helps bring out my masculine side." Many men who perform rhythmic gymnastics insist they are different from women gymnasts by claiming their bodies are different (Chimot and Louveau 2010). Some male dancers, like Denny, suggest men and women are built differently and have unique muscles. These men believe that similar movements look different depending on the sex of the body executing them. "That is one of the reasons, and one of the big reasons, it is important to have those males in there (belly dance perfor-mances) just because of the difference in the same move," Denny claims. Denny uses tools in belly dance to showcase masculinity. Studies examining masculine

29

leisure suggest that men treat leisure pursuits as arenas in which they reaffirm traditional masculinity (Hunt 2004; Schwalbe 1996). For example, skydiving, a predominantly masculine activity, supports male dominance, risk taking, and "hyperheterosexuality" (Anderson and Taylor, 2010). Similarly, gun collectors draw from traditional cowboy images and perform masculinity by displaying technical knowledge and skills associated with gun ownership (Anderson and Taylor, 2010).

Mark and I discuss his experience in flamenco compared to belly dance. When he studied flamenco, his instructor advised him against using his hips. However, he enjoys performing hip movements. Mark left flamenco partly because he didn't like the strict guidelines that he felt dictated how men and women should dance. But in belly dance, "I haven't experienced any guidelines with gender," he explains. He postulates that the lack of gendered instruction "might have to do with the American Tribal Style" of dance in which he participates. "I feel like it's a tribe. We're all in it together. It doesn't matter who you are. The same rules apply to everyone," Mark comments about the universal arm movements, hand gestures, and cues that are used by all ATS dancers. As he suggests, the codification and structured nature of ATS is more universal and dancers such as Mark view it as less gendered, and therefore feel less of a need to "masculinize" the dance compared to other forms of belly dance. Mark is one of the few males with whom I spoke who did not work to masculinize belly dance. ATS may be less threatening to men because both men and women construct it as representing strength, power, and being grounded. Therefore, ATS may be constructed as more in line with traditional notions of masculinity.

Like Mark, Phil is another ATS male belly dancer who is less concerned with masculinizing the dance. "We're all doing the exact same movement, and I don't distinguish a tall man or short man or tall woman or short woman because it's all going to look different." He insists that men and women do the same movements given the standardized ATS vocabulary. "I might push my hip a little bigger because [the women in his group] have full hips." Phil wants his hip movements to look as large as his tribe members. However, he reiterates, "I do not have to masculinize my movements in ATS because I consider it almost inherent in the movements." The strength and lifted posture "satisfies any [masculinity] issues I could have."

Although Phil does not feel a need to masculinize his participation in ATS, he felt very different when he first got involved in belly dance and danced Egyptian Orientale style belly dance. "When I dance, I don't want to look like a coquette, a cute young lady who is very flirty . . . I'm a big old man. I can't do cute." Phil's description of looking coquettish mirrors Cameron's earlier comments about some dancers being "coy." Phil stands up from the large over-sized chair in which he sits and overly exaggerates a little girl. He contracts his body bringing his hands close to his face and does a curtsey. I immediately start laughing. "You are laughing, and it looks stupid on me. Look at me, I'm so cute," Phil says as he mimics the high-pitched voice of a young girl. Phil tells me about a time he danced at an Egyptian wedding and he heard something "cute" in the music. "I heard this in the music and thought 'I need to masculinize this.' I held my arms differently and my posture back a little bit. So I did the same technical move, but I thought I needed to project a more masculine version of it because it's not coquette." Phil begins to show me different movements. "Instead of being all cute, I brought my arms down to here [chest height], which is a little more rigid. Same move, but stronger. Arms out to the side. It's a guy showing off his muscles. This is me flexing," he says as he tightens his right bicep.

Early on in his dance practice, one of Phil's teacher said to him, "I am guessing you are doing that [emphasizing masculinity] because you are afraid of looking like a girl." His teacher reminded him that no one is going to mistake him for a girl. Having a large, stocky build gives Phil a degree of built-in masculinity, which, along with dancing the American Tribal Style, may offer him some freedom from feeling the need to assert masculinity through dance.

"Cabaret is mainly feminine movements, while tribal has masculine movements built in to it because it's a bit more earthy," Henry explains to me. For both men and women, these constructs of different dance styles have real consequences for how participants view them, which influences their preferred styles. Along with tribal styles, Henry also likes Turkish folkloric dance that he describes as more "grounded" as opposed to Turkish Orientale, which he says is more similar to Egyptian Orientale. He tells me that cabaret dancing is derived more from Turkish and Egyptian Orientale, while tribal dance is rooted more in Turkish folkloric dance. "Soft movements tend to be more feminine. Sharp movements tend to have more power and tend to be considered more masculine," Henry tells me. "Things that are earthy tend to be more masculine and things that are airy tend to be more feminine. One of the reasons I'm drawn toward tribal is most of its vocabulary is based on Turkish dance, which is more earthy, so I get a more inspiration form that because it's easier for me," he explains.

Gender is relational. Female is in relation to male, and male is in relation to female (Buchbinder 2013). As Henry demonstrates, when dancers talk about masculinizing movements, they distinguish the masculine from the feminine. One reason why Henry may desire to separate his masculine dance from feminine movements is that, unlike Phil, Henry is shorter and more slender. His body type does not project the built-in stereotypical masculine features that Phil's taller and larger frame exudes. Therefore, along with dancing a slightly different style than Phil, Henry may also have to work to masculinize movements given his smaller stature.

31

"My hands were too soft. I had feminine hands"

Men who participate in female-dominated activities may be particularly moti-vated to express their masculinity in ways that adhere to culturally accepted standards of what it means to be a man. For instance, young men who partici-pate in the "feminine" sport of rhythmic gymnastics actively work to construct their identity as men. These men experience pressure from family members and peers to adhere to typical masculine ideals (Chimot and Louveau 2010). Likewise, male cheerleaders attempt to "save face" by cheering in hypermas-culine ways (Bemiller 2005). Furthermore, male tango and ballet dancers emphasize macho aspects of their respective dances to counteract effeminate stereotyping of the dance (Fisher 2009; Tobin 1998).

Similar to male rhythmic gymnasts, cheerleaders, and tango and ballet dancers, many of the men with whom I spoke work to masculinize belly dance movements. The desire to masculinize a movement suggests that its default is feminine. I did not speak to any female dancers who suggested that they desired to make a movement more feminine. Jeffrey Tobin (1998) dis-cusses how some male tango dancers consider it effeminate to put too much effort into their moves. Therefore, male dancers take a minimalist approach to leading and strive to showcase the women. To draw too much attention to their own moves is considered too feminine. In other words, effort is emas-culating. It is acceptable for men to have natural talent, but appearing as if they are trying too hard may lessen the extent to which they are perceived as masculine men. Likewise, some male belly dancers perform particular moves, execute movements in specific ways, and avoid some movements to resist appearing effeminate.

Throughout our lengthy phone call, Andy and I talk about his experiences as a man in belly dance. "I'm very masculine when I dance," Andy replies when I ask him to describe the type of dance he participates in. "There's nothing feminine about what I do," he continues. He claims that the basic movements that men and women do can be similar, but "I don't do them in feminine ways." "How do you dance masculine?" I inquire. "It's all in how you hold yourself, and how you project yourself," Andy explains with the confidence one would expect from someone who has been involved in the dance for over thirty-five years. "The others just look like they are imitating women. They have learned too much of the modern cabaret style of dance," Andy explains, distancing himself from other male dancers whom he claims dance like women. "I don't do all the flittery flowy fingers. When I do an arm wave or undulation, it fol-lows all the way through to my fingers, but it never goes limp." Andy refers to some Egyptian hand movements that appear as if one is petting a cat. "Some of the men doing that is like 'Eww!' No no no!" Andy exclaims. About how he dances, Andy continues, "You're up and your back is straight and your arms are strong and not wobbly and hold your fingers like a man. When I dance most of the time my palms are up and facing in toward my body. I do things with my hands. They don't go weak. They always stay really strong."

"All the men in Egypt I've met, they dance, but they don't dance like women," Andy says as he continues distinguishing between male and female dancers. When Andy first saw a video of one particular Egyptian dancer, he thought, "Wow! Praise the lord! He's Egyptian and dances just like I do! He's a very masculine man!" "What was so masculine about him?" I inquire. "He dances with a lot of rivato, with force behind him. It's very grounded. Although he can be light at times, he dances right into the ground." Andy continues explaining how this Egyptian man's dancing is very similar to his own when he says, "I feel I am very connected to the ground except when I'm spinning, but I spin just above the ground. You're so connected to the earth." Here, Andy draws from some Egyptian male dancers as exemplars of masculinity.

Early in his dance experience, Henry was approached by a woman after he had finished some social dancing. "You were taught by a girl," Henry recalls this woman saying to him. Confused by how this stranger could have known the gender of Henry's teacher just by watching him dance, he pushed for more information. "My hands were too soft. I had a very feminine hands," Henry explains. He demonstrates a masculine hand by straightening his fingers and placing them together. He contrasts this "masculine" hand with a "feminine" hand displaying slightly bent and softer fingers. Along with holding the hands a certain way, Henry explains how hip shimmies can be made more masculine or feminine. "A soft shimmy can be feminine where a very hard glute shimmy can be masculine and more powerful. Having that dichotomy of sharp versus smooth can make something more masculine or feminine," Henry says, echoing how some female dancers liken their soft movements to being "graceful."

Henry has taken workshops, both cabaret and the American Tribal Style, with several male dancers. However, he did not feel like any of these workshops emphasized masculine technique in dance. Because developing a masculine style is so important to him, he created his own masculine technique through trial and error by scrutinizing his video-taped performances and studying other dance forms that he says distinguish between masculine and feminine movements, such as Indian dance. He also borrows movements from female flamenco dancers that he says are "powerful" and can be used to portray masculinity. I wonder why portraying masculinity in his dance is so important to Henry. "I identify as very masculine . . . so it's much easier for me to portray masculine form," he replies. I ask Henry how he is masculine. "Femininity is more creativity and masculinity is more action." In belly dance, this difference translates into bigger movements. "I connect power and strength to masculinity whereas softness and protection to femininity."

33

Kevin isn't performing belly dance much when we meet. "Once I have my technique down, it might be a different story. It's the male dances. If I was going to do the female stuff, I'd need to . . . masculinize it and [work on my] technique using the hips or chest, and undulations. I want to do it right," he says. "Masculinizing the dance would look like what?" I wonder. Kevin explains:

> Men are strong and powerful. You don't let your wrists go easy. It's OK to be graceful . . . Men are hard. It's just a matter of how you hold your arms and stuff. It makes a difference. You don't want to be doing these feminine things with the audience unless you have a big old grin and make it look like it's a big old joke. Other things I've heard is you want sharper movements, bigger movements. You're supposed to be doing this as being powerful. There's a lot more jumping involved. That's a big man thing. My knees can't handle that. You are going from a jump right down into the ground and right back up. Very athletic because we are trying to show our power and all that stuff. If you watch some of the cane dances on YouTube, they do quite a bit of jumping. They are athletic, showing off their power, their strength. Women are showing off: "I'm pretty. I'm beautiful."

Kevin implies that being graceful is more associated with femininity, as he continues talking about how men should be "hard." He suggests that men should only perform like female dancers if they are kidding and being playful with the audience. Joking around and using humor suggests that it is undesirable to transgress gender boundaries. At the same time, the poking fun can be viewed as derogatory or demeaning femininity. Joking relieves pressure or expectations to reaffirm one's masculinity because it isn't actually leaving masculinity. Therefore, the potential threat to masculinity is diminished (Kimmel 2008). In "Dude, You're a Fag," Pascoe (2011) shows that boys invoke the fag by exaggerating femininity and pretending to be desirable to other boys. By imitation, they assure others that they are not gay and assume masculinity immediately after their humorous performance. They mock exaggerated femininity and desirability to assure themselves and others they are heterosexual. Finally, Kevin hints at messages that he has received from other people, most likely instructors, about how to masculinize belly dance, and he takes these messages as appropriate guidelines for his dance. If he cannot adhere to these guidelines, he is not comfortable performing in public.

Dance teachers occasionally use gendered language and instruction to emphasize masculine behavior, such as gestures and movement execution that they believe fall in line with typical notions of masculinity (Risner 2009). Many belly dance instructors, primarily women, reinforce gender boundaries. Brooke shows videos of men and women dancing during some of her classes. She says, "I teach [men in her classes] to dance like a man and not like a woman.""What are some of the differences?" I wonder. "I ask him to change it to be more masculine. I ask him to show me strength in certain areas where a woman would not," Brooke says.

Brooke's approach to teaching men dance reminds me of how one of my early teachers instructed a male to dance. Our instructor commented that female and male dancers should hold their hands differently. Women were asked to keep their fingers straight out, while the men were told to make fists (see Figure 2.1). Therefore, not only do some male dancers attempt to masculinize belly dance, some female instructors reinforce the same expectations regarding technique.

Dancing bodies often highlight traditional notions of masculine and feminine and can be heavily divided by gender in terms of movement and placement. For instance, men may take up a different physical space on a stage (Albright 1997). Along with teaching men to masculinize dance movements, some instructors assign men to play stereotypical masculine roles in belly dance acts. For instance, a group might create an act that tells a story of a sultan and his dancers. Men are typically asked to play the role of a sultan, while his dancers are played by women. Denny assumed a particular role in a group sword dance because his troupe wanted a man to play the part. Denny's instructor thought that one of the sword dances would create a feeling of "grrr and that testosterone," he tells me. When women dance, it is "very beautiful, but the sword dance is like a march. It is very militant," Denny continues. His instructor thought that "a male could portray it very well. So, she put me in there." Similar to assigning men and women to assume traditional gender roles in a belly dance performance, the heteronormativity embedded in ballroom dance is emphasized with the male–female pairing of dance partners (Marion 2008).

"I'm not wearing a female costume"

Male dancers use costumes to distinguish themselves from women. "I'm not wearing a female costume," Phil tells me. Rather than the skirts and coin bras that female American Tribal Style dancers wear, Phil has a coin vest. "I want to stay as true to the ATS uniform as possible, so I wear a choli, but I don't wear a bra because a bra is a female thing," Phil continues. Furthermore, Phil does not wear skirts because he sees no reason to wear one and "it also makes me look like a female, and I don't want to do that." Although he does not feel a need to masculinize ATS moves, he uses costuming to "stay in the male." As part of his masculine ATS costuming, Phil also wears a turban. "The turban is a big one. Traditionally in Eastern culture, men will have the turbans."

Male ballet dancers frequently wear tights (Fisher 2009), while male belly dancers are surrounded by women dressed in skirts and decorated bras, and

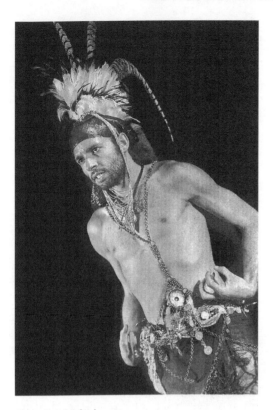

Figure 2.1 Male dancer

Photo credit: Carrie Meyer/The Dancers Eye.

occasionally showing their midriffs. Male belly dancers also have to manage frustrations that accompany a dearth of male costuming that they think is appropriate for them. As we wrap up our chat, I ask Denny if there is anything that he does not like about belly dance or that he finds frustrating. Without hesitation, he replies:

> That I can't find male outfits on the rack. It sounds kind of frivolous, but it is frustrating. I have to make most of my outfits or have somebody else make them for me. You can go to certain stores or places in the mall and you will find outfits for girls . . . You can even go to Goodwill and find tops and pants that go well for girls. Very rarely am I able to find harem pants or things of the like for guys. If they do have harem pants, they go up to a size thirteen or something. I don't wear that size, I am not a girl.

Much like Denny, Henry also has difficulty finding costumes for men, so he sews many of his costumes. Some people may find it ironic that dancers like

Henry engage in the stereotypically feminine activity of sewing in order to have costumes that they feel are sufficiently masculine. However, several male dancers believe that sewing their own costumes is the only way for them to acquire a belly dance wardrobe in which they feel comfortable. As we were discussing one of his costume pieces, Henry stated that:

> If you walk through a marketplace, you will not see many outfits for male belly dancers I find flattering. Occasionally I can find a unisex vest. It's not very often I find costumes with pants. These pants I made (he gestures toward the pantaloons he is wearing during our talk) . . . I have to make my own costumes.

Similar to Phil and other male dancers, Henry's typical costume consists of pantaloons or silk wrap pants, a vest, a head scarf, and multiple items for his hips, such as scarves, a panel belt, and a tassel belt. "Sometimes I'll wear a coin belt, but never the triangular sash. The triangle is more feminine. The triangle represents the V of the woman's pelvis," he tells me. Henry will wear a straight belt rather than one that is curved. Choosing to wear a straight belt rather than a triangular hip scarf is one way Henry uses costumes to display masculinity.

"I do male Middle Eastern dance"

Some male dancers linguistically separate themselves from female dancers by avoiding the term "belly dancer." When men dance tango with other men, they do not refer to it as "dancing," but rather "practicing" (Tobin 1998). These linguistic devices function to emphasize masculinity and avoid being placed in the same category as women. Like some other contemporary male Middle Eastern dancers (Saleem 2009), several times throughout our conversation Nick reiterates that he does not belly dance. He tells me about men in Egypt who dance with swords or who folk dance to celebrate a harvest. "That's the big distinction between traditional dancing that Middle Eastern men could do that was considered socially acceptable and the men that did belly dancing. I don't do belly dancing." "What would you say you do?" I ask. "I do Middle Eastern male dance, which is a different animal than Middle Eastern female dance, which is known today as belly dance," Nick succinctly replies.

As we finish our conversation, I ask Nick if there is anything else he wants to add. "The main thing I wanted to make sure we touched on: I'm not a belly dancer," he reiterates. Nick's insistence that he is not a "belly dancer" is a fine example of role distance, i.e. the gap between how we enact a role and the obligations associated with that role (Goffman 1961). Separating ourselves from part of a role that we dislike allows us to fulfill some obligations of the role while maintaining our self-respect (Stebbins 1969). Insisting that he is not a belly dancer, but performs another kind of dance allows Nick to participate in this community without being associated with a "female" dance, thereby ensuring that he is not confused with other male dancers who may dance like women. Not only does Nick suggest there is a difference in how he moves, but also in what the dance represents and he wants everyone to understand that the meaning he attaches to the dance is different to how he perceives female belly dance.

Adhering to traditional notions of masculinity can be advantageous for male dancers in the United States. Men hold a privileged position in multiple forms of dance and their relative scarcity gives them an advantage (Mennesson 2009). Andy was a professional dancer for decades. "I danced in clubs making an incredible salary because I was a traditional male belly dancer," he tells me. Dancing in nightclubs, Andy made "[the same amount of money] I would be making if I worked for a big corporation." He could demand $150 for one twenty-minute show, "and they'd say OK no problem," Andy remembers. However, the female dancers may earn only $25 for the entire evening. "I had quite a career. I totally supported myself dancing," Andy tells me. His novelty as a male dancer intrigued the general public. He appeared on television shows, and in magazines and newspapers. Andy's experiences are similar to some male ballroom dancers who are valued for their scarcity and experience less competition for jobs (Fisher 2009; Marion 2008). These dynamics in ballroom and belly dance echo the experiences of men in female-dominated workplaces, such as nursing, elementary school teaching, and social work, who may find themselves placed on a "glass escalator." In other words, they can become more successful and more quickly than some of their female counterparts partly due to the fact that as men, they are a valued oddity in that profession (Schrock and Schwalbe 2009; Williams 1992).

Gendering belly dance

To varying degrees, both men and women use belly dance to construct masculinities and femininities. They do so in similar ways using similar tools, but strive for different outcomes. Dancers play with different styles, costumes, bodily adornments, and movements to demonstrate masculinity and femininity. Male dancers strategically choose costumes, use verbal descriptors, and emphasize particular movements to display their masculinity. Men also believe that some styles of belly dance are more conducive to stereotypical displays of masculinity. Men who perform styles that they believe are more in line with traditional notions of manhood are less concerned about presenting a hypermasculine dance compared to men who perform styles that they associate with stereotypical notions of femininity.

Men take up more public space than women, and are more willing to violate women's space and interrupt the talk of women (Henley 1986). For some female participants, belly dance is a space away from other areas of their lives where they do not have opportunities to play with traditional notions of femininity. Belly dance, particularly the costumes and accessories, offers women tools to play with hyperfemininity. At the same time, different belly dance styles offer a variety of tools and linguistic anchors to construct different types of femininity.

In front of the sea of 160 students in my sociology of gender class I discuss the constructed nature of gender and how notions of masculinity and femininity can change over time. "I think I've become more girlie as I've gotten older," I announce to my class. "Maybe it's the belly dancing," I add.

Note

1 One important exception is the presence of live musicians, who, based on my years of observation, tend to be mostly (but not all) men. I have only seen musicians at performances, rehearsals, and drum circles, but not at regular instructional classes or workshops (unless it is a drum workshop). Although men attend the public events at which some belly dancers perform, the gender composition of audience members varies by performance context, restaurants or shows.

Chapter 3

The belly dancing body

First let's be honest with ourselves. We are never going to win the commercial beauty game. The reality is many clients want the movie star look. They buy into the fantasy of perfection and want the pretty face. Many of us will never have the type of "pretty privilege" that will land us the expensive gigs and opportunities. That is ok. This is about coming to terms with the fact that while mainstream beauty ideals still apply to this art form for certain marketing purposes; they do not define the true beauty of our art. The depth of beauty in the belly dance community is broader and richer than the surface of any Hollywood ideal.

(Hayam 2015)

The above excerpt is taken from an online article written by a belly dancer about body image and how norms regarding the body within belly dance circles are influenced by wider cultural ideals. Hayam expresses her belief that dancers should stay true to what she believes belly dance represents. It is striking that this post circulates through various belly dance communities suggesting that (1) dancers generally agree with the ideas expressed in this post and (2) they want other belly dancers to share Hayam's feelings. In this chapter, I explore body reflexivity and how dancers evaluate themselves depending on their audiences. To this end, I analyze messages about the body that are typically shared within belly dance communities and those that are highly contested. Furthermore I consider how wider cultural expectations within the United States influence internal messages.

Body reflexivity

All of us have bodies and all of us are bodies (Crossley 2005; Turner 1984). Our bodies are situated in everyday life meaning that we experience the world through our senses by interpreting what happens around us. Waskul and Vannini (2006:3) define embodiment as, "the process by which the object-body is actively experienced, produced, sustained, and/or transformed as a subject-body." The body, self, and interaction are all interrelated and each influences the other (Waskul and van der Riet 2002). As such, the body is both an object and subject (Crossley 2005). As an object, we have a physical tangible body that is put on display and is seen by others. Our bodies are also subjects as we experience and attach meaning to them (Waskul 2003). When we act toward our bodies as both object and subject, we reinforce Mead's (1934) concepts of the "I" (active agent who is performing the action) and "me" (passive object receiving the action of the "I").

We are rooted in groups and our experiences are shaped by the contexts in which we are located. If we seek approval or love from those with whom we interact, we are motivated to monitor and alter our bodies and behaviors in the hope of receiving affirmation. Borrowing from Charles Horton Cooley's idea of the "looking glass self" (1983 [1902]:151–152), Waskul and Vannini (2006:5) coined the term the "looking-glass body" referring to how we evaluate our bodies based on how (we imagine) others perceive us. Likewise, when we gaze on other bodies, we make judgments, and the people on whom we gaze imagine our evaluations. Crossley (2006c:1) refers to this process as "reflexive embodiment," which he defines as the "tendency to perceive, emote about, reflect and act upon one's own body." In other words, people generally have some understanding about how others perceive them.

We attempt to manage how other people view us through bodily adornments and modifications. As Waskul (2003:72) states, "It is in how we uniquely manipulate and configure relationships between the appearance of our body as an object and the experience of our body as a subject that we achieve a distinct embodied self." In other words, the body-object is decorated and altered as we experience our bodies in social interaction. Crossley (2005, 2006b) identifies several reflexive body techniques that people use to present their bodies while attempting to influence how they are perceived. Examples include brushing one's hair and teeth and cosmetic surgery. Reflexive body techniques support group identities and signify group boundaries. For instance, Scott (2010) shows that how swimmers move and treat their bodies illustrates an individual desire to stay fit. At the same time, their bodily movements influence how they are perceived by others.

Dance participants primarily consist of instructors and students. In the Brazilian dance and martial art *capoeira*, instructor bodies are typically admired and their appearance and/or abilities are aspired to by the students as students observe teachers' movements and attempt to replicate those same steps (Stephens and Delamont 2006). Likewise, one belly dancer constantly watches her instructor's feet "in the hopes that someday my feet will be her feet," Jordan remarks. Like practitioners of *capoeira*, belly dancers spend hours, days, years, and sometimes decades practicing and perfecting bodily dance movements and refining their dance skills to achieve desired ideals.

Uncontested internal bodily messages

Many norms within belly dance center on how dancers should view and treat their bodies. Most of these messages are generally uncontested, while others spark great controversy. Dancers generally agree that belly dance is a beneficial and enjoyable form of physical exercise that is available to bodies of varying abilities, shapes, sizes, and ages. In other words, there is wide affirmation that belly dance is overtly body-positive in that people with a variety of bodies are accepted and welcomed in belly dance.

> If you want to start loving your body, teach it to move in ways you never thought it could.
> (Plus Size Bellydancers/Dangerous Curves Facebook page)

Royce (2002:3) defines dance as "the body making patterns in time and space." Since the body is the center of any dance form dancers necessarily become more aware of their bodies, gain bodily knowledge, and develop more confidence (Shay 2008). Many dancers claim that belly dance increases their endurance, muscle tone, posture, coordination, cardiovascular health, and, to varying degrees, flexibility. Belly dance also encourages participants to move their bodies in unique and interesting ways, resulting in greater appreciation for their physical forms. In this way, belly dance is similar to running (Altheide and Pfuhl 1980) in that one strong motivation for participating in both activities is beneficial transformation of the body.

The core movements of belly dance, such as isolating the hips and torso, differ from other dance forms, such as ballet or ballroom. Belly dance emphasizes parts of the body that many Westerners are not accustomed to moving. Learning new movements and how they fit together renders belly dance unique compared to other forms of exercise, such as running, going to the gym, or taking an aerobics class. As a result, dancers appreciate their bodies' abilities, meet the challenges of learning something new, and gain confidence from the experiences. Like runners (Altheide and Pfuhl 1980), accomplishing the physical goals of belly dance contributes to positive changes in one's attitude toward self. For instance, Trisha tells me, "I am learning to move my body in different ways, so I am enjoying this a lot more. I tried aerobics, I am not a jogger, and I don't like to swim." Like Trisha, many dancers participate in this activity because they do not enjoy other forms of physical exercise, yet similar to people who run (Altheide and Pfuhl 1980) and those who join gyms (Crossley 2006a), many dancers got involved in the activity because they wanted to be more physically active.

Engaging in physical activities helps women feel a sense of accomplishment and supports their self-esteem (Chrisler and Lamont 2002), and this may be particularly true for people who engage in highly gendered activities. For instance, people who participate in burlesque experience empowerment, greater confidence, and increased self-esteem (Regehr 2012). Belly dancers similarly feel pride and excitement when they perform a movement correctly or master some technique. "Is there anything you get from belly dance that you don't get any place else," I ask Joni. "The self-satisfaction that you get when you are trying to learn a new choreography or something of that nature and you finally get it," she replies. "I finally got it. I did it. That was good. I am proud of myself," she exclaims. Similar to runners (Altheide and Pfuhl 1980) and people who join gyms (Crossley 2006a), the vast majority of belly dancers get involved in the activity through personal motivation (rather than a doctor persuading them to take up the activity) and the decision to do so is rooted in concerns about their life, appearance, and physical ability.

"I can actually work out without hurting myself"

Since the new millennium, Americans have tried a myriad of tactics to create fit and healthy bodies, such as various workouts and diets. Individuals are held accountable for their health and fitness, and cultural expectations dictate that people should engage in health-inducing behaviors. Those who do not are viewed as socially irresponsible, immoral, and lazy (Edgley 2006).

Some belly dancers manage chronic physical and mental health conditions that prevent them from engaging in other forms of exercise. However, their lived experiences with various health challenges heighten their awareness of bodily limitations and their desire for exercise. These dancers can participate in belly dance despite their physical challenges. Because people are generally expected to be healthy and engage in health-enhancing behaviors, achieving that ideal can be difficult for people whose bodies do not function as well as other bodies. People with less able bodies are subject to stigma, or ridicule, for not living up to societal standards (Goffman 1963). Finding a physical activity that one can engage in can lessen feelings of stigmatization. In this sense, belly dance allows dancers to participate in Western norms of "healthism," or health-enhancing activities, such as exercise (Crawford 1980).

In many ways belly dance is both forgiving of limitations and easier on dancers' bodies compared to other physical pursuits. For example, belly dance is the only physical activity in which Maggie can participate. Although only in her twenties, Maggie manages nerve issues and has a rare joint disease that does not allow her to be very physically active. She cannot use elliptical machines or participate in low impact forms of exercise due to her extensive nerve challenges. At times she experiences numbness in her legs and feet. "Belly dance is literally about the only thing I can do," Maggie says. It helps her joints feel better, whereas other forms of exercise aggravate her joints. One of the largest challenges with Maggie's condition is she needs to have strong muscles. "I got really lucky finding this because I actually can work out without hurting myself," Maggie explains.

Charmaz and Rosenfeld (2006) suggest that people with chronic illnesses and disabilities experience a tension between their body, self, and identity to a greater degree than those who do not live with such disabilities. Compared to those with more able bodies, people with disabilities and other physical challenges may be even more self-conscious as they work to overcome physical limitations. Belly dance helps Maggie maintain some mastery over her body and some degree of physical capability. For some dancers with physical limitations, such as Maggie, belly dance is one tool they use to both maintain and enhance their bodies' capabilities. As one dancer commented, "If I don't dance, I can't walk."

Although both men and women value belly dance as a form of exercise, women attach meaning to additional aspects within belly dance, while men suggest that exercise is one of the primary reasons they participate in belly dance. Perhaps doing so brings men's participation in the dance more in line with traditional notions of masculinity, much like male swimmers who define their participation as primarily a form of exercise (Scott 2010). Some male dancers tell me that belly dance gives them energy to survive long working days that are sometimes combined with the responsibilities of being a college student. Furthermore, like Maggie, some men find that the dance helps them address various physical ailments.

Kevin joined belly dance classes about a year after he collapsed due to working two full-time jobs and attending college full-time. As part of his recovery, "I started thinking I need to do something physical," he recalls. Kevin tried some physical education and dance classes, which eventually led him to belly dance. Belly dance "requires more work, so I kind of feel like it's the most effective form [of dance] to take," Kevin says. Kevin reflected on his failing health and concluded that he needed to become more physically active. He pursued belly dance because he believed that the additional "work" would help him recover from his earlier exhaustion.

"For me, definitely exercise," Larry quickly responds to my inquiry about the benefits he receives from belly dance. "Just getting out and doing something and giving me something to look forward to every week," he continues. Along with wanting to remain physically active, Larry has dealt with overextended tendons in his shoulders. His participation in belly dance has helped mitigate his shoulder discomfort. "Before I started belly dance, I definitely felt a sense of joint pain and stuff like that, and I honestly don't feel anything like that [anymore]," Larry comments since getting involved in belly dance about a year earlier. Although he is only in his mid-twenties, Larry also has trouble with his knees and weak ankles. "But now they are actually getting stronger," he tells me. "The benefits for me have just been improving my body and making me more proud of it," Larry says. As Larry suggests, being physically active through belly dance and improving one's physical health and comfort can help people develop more positive feelings toward their bodies.

"I've struggled with body image a lot of my life"

Memes are posted on Facebook stating that "vigilant tribal husky hates it when any dancer tries to body shame another dancer." Sharing these phrases sends powerful messages regarding acceptable ways that dancers should act toward each other. In my over thirteen years of experience in multiple belly dance communities, aside from the rare story of instructors who only accept students whose appearance approximates a standard Western ideal of attractiveness, I have never heard dancers directly chided for their physical appearance. It is possible that comments to the contrary are made in more private settings. If this is the case, it reiterates that it is unacceptable to publicly body shame another dancer. Advertisements and posters with phrases such as "Love your belly" and "Bellybration" (an amalgamation of celebration and belly) are used to encourage people to register for dance classes. These signs and rhetoric suggest strong norms that participants should feel proud of their bodies and work toward acceptance.

Belly dance helps both male and female dancers feel better about their bodies. As he alluded to earlier, belly dance helps increase Larry's body image. When he was growing up, his brother was verbally abusive. "You live 18 years of your life being told how worthless you are," Larry recalls. But, with belly dance, "I feel great!" Larry exclaims. "I like the way it makes me feel about my body," he continues. Before he got involved in the dance, Larry felt like he had a "beer gut type thing going on, but now I'm like 'Oh man, this thing is gorgeous!'"

"I think for me, one of the most powerful gifts it gave me was learning to love my body," Mark says about the benefits he receives from belly dance. "As a gay man, I know I'm surrounded by images of men with six packs and this completely idealized masculine form. I feel like for the longest time, I did not have that body," he continues. Before he entered high school, Mark says he was a little overweight. He eventually lost a lot of weight, but claims he did so through unhealthy means. "I developed minor anorexia. I just stopped eating. My mental process in how I viewed my body was very negative," Mark recalls. "I think belly dance really forced me to get in touch with my body and how beautiful my body is no matter what shape and size it is. So that's been a powerful gift belly dance has given me," he says.

Along with some male dancers, many female participants use belly dance to help them develop and/or continue a positive relationship with their body. Some belly dance writers suggest that appearing more "womanly" and curvaceous is preferable to a thin body (Dallal 2004). When a woman enters a belly dance class, she most likely sees various body shapes, sizes, and ages that range from short to tall, skinny to voluptuous, and young to mature. No matter how a woman looks, chances are she will find someone who has a comparable appearance in a belly dance class. Seeing someone in a class that has a similar build can help a participant feel more at ease with her own body and less concerned about whether her classmates will accept her. A participant looks at other dancers who share her physical features and sees how attractive and capable they look dancing. She may reason that if other dancers can look good, so can she.

Viewing women of multiple shapes, sizes, and ages is a welcome break from the narrow images of beauty with which we are bombarded on a daily basis. This is especially true when the activity involves highly visible bodily displays. Dance presentations provide ample opportunity for (hopefully positive) feedback and affirmation of one's appearance (Albright 1997). Belly dance helps women confront cultural norms about ideal body appearance (Moe 2011). Participating in belly dance and receiving positive feedback from fellow dancers and audience members about their appearance and dance performances boosts their self-esteem.

"How do you feel about your body?" I ask Emma. Although she appears smaller than the average American woman, "I've struggled with body image a lot of my life," Emma tells me. Her father had a very powerful, yet negative, effect on how Emma views her body. "One of the reasons I think he left my mom is because she gained weight," Emma surmises. When she was younger, her father "sat my sister and I both down and said that we both needed to lose weight otherwise our husbands would leave us," Emma recalls. Partly as a result of her father's statements, Emma struggled with bulimia for a few years while she was in college.

Along with body shape and size diversity, many dancers appreciate that the activity welcomes people throughout the life span. In a culture where aging can be difficult, especially for women (Clarke 2011), belly dance provides an outlet for some people to feel comfortable in their aging bodies. An older body challenges culturally accepted standards of beauty, which can threaten a women's sense of self and femininity (Clarke 2011). The aging female body is sometimes judged as ugly and undesirable (Holstein 2006; Wolf 1990).

When Kylie first got involved in the activity, she found "beautiful women my age trying to express themselves and be joyful and not be self-conscious," she tells me. In her fifties, Kylie feels inspired and at home around "bright and beautiful women who are strong," despite a few gray hairs and wrinkling that accompany the natural aging process. "It's not ugly! It's beautiful!" Kylie exclaims. In belly dance, Kylie finds kindred spirits who share her belief that "despite what we see on television," wrinkling skin and gray hairs are attractive. Some dancers believe that belly dance is accessible for women of all ages because it is based on natural movement. Women of all ages, including those with aging bodies (much like people with physical limitations), may not risk injury to the extent that they would with other physical activities and dance forms.

Whether it is related to ability, weight, and/or age, many dancers develop a more positive view of their bodies in belly dance partly by receiving affirmation from audiences. Although she used to see herself as "skinny," Grace tells me that she is now "a big girl." Despite viewing herself as a larger woman, "I still get just as many compliments," she tells me about the positive feedback she receives from patrons. Although people enjoy and admire her dancing, Grace admits that she occasionally engages in the same damaging self-talk as some other dancers. "I know when I look in the mirror I think the same thing as everyone else. I'm fat. I'm overweight. I'm forty-seven years old. Who am I trying to kid?" she tells me. However, dancing and feeling positive energy from the audience helps Grace quiet the negativity.

This dynamic of improving one's body image due to praise from others is not unlike people who display their nude bodies via webcam (Waskul 2002). Although the particular settings are quite different and belly dancers are not nude, in both cases, the body is both an acting subject and viewed object during interaction. Webcam cybersex participants and belly dancers put their bodies "out there" to be viewed by others. People at the other end of the webcam or in the audience subjectively gaze on the bodies and evaluate what they see. Some cybersex participants do not feel that their partners physically desire them and they become dissatisfied with their bodies. However, displaying their bodies over the Internet and engaging in webcam sex with people who praise and compliment their appearance helps them feel sexy, desirable, and attractive (Waskul 2002). Likewise, many belly dancers who received disapproving messages from their families and feel ashamed of their appearance as a result, begin to assess their bodies more positively through their experiences with belly dance. In both settings, people become "re-enchanted" (Waskul 2002) and discover a renewed sense of appreciation for their body.

"Belly dancing is the celebration of jiggle"

Rather than hiding one's fat and feeling ashamed, dancers occasionally redefine having extra weight on their body as something positive. Although Bess is very slender and tall compared to the average American woman, belly dance helps her feel a little better about some parts of her figure that she does not like "because it is OK to have a stomach if you are a belly dancer." "You don't have to have this perfect body that is this ideal we have in America," she explains. Bess says belly dancers "can still look really great if you don't live up to that ideal." Bess shares a story about a time she returned home after a belly dance class during which the students learned shimmies. She exclaimed to her mother that "belly dancing is the celebration of jiggle!" Regardless of her small frame, Bess has clearly incorporated the body-affirming messages she has received from other members of the community.

Joy does not consider herself skinny and she elects to perform with her stomach exposed rather than covering it with a body stocking. She adorns her body in a standard American cabaret costume consisting of a decorated bra and skirt. "Seeing the flesh jiggle is such a beautiful, powerful part of it, and it's so amazing," Joy tells me. Joy belly danced at her son's elementary school for an international event and "So many mothers come up to me afterwards to tell me how beautiful I am and how I make them feel so much better. I make them feel like they can be that beautiful too because I have a real woman's body, and I'm using it." Much like dancers who gaze upon other dancers and judge themselves positively, audience members watch Joy dance with an exposed stomach, which increases their self-esteem. Joy believes that wearing belly dance costumes and revealing one's middle accentuates a dancer's beauty.

It is not uncommon for female dancers to tell me that the most attractive pictures they have of themselves are in their dance costumes, and it is not infrequent that they post these pictures on the Internet. "It's pretty," Julia tells me about using a picture of her belly dancing as her Facebook profile picture. "People see pictures of me dancing and are like 'oh my gosh you're so beautiful,'" she continues. People praising her appearance in belly dance costumes enhances Julia's self-image. "In my day to day life, I don't get fancy. So, I don't have a lot of fancy pictures of myself other than my wedding and dancing," she tells me. It is customary for tribal style dancers, such as Julia, to heavily adorn their bodies, paint their faces, and style their hair when they dance. Similar to Jorgensen's (2006) study of tribal dancers, many participants with whom I spoke feel the costumes are flattering and appealing. Costumes can enhance how a dancer evaluates her appearance and how outsiders judge her attractiveness. As one dancer in a costume before a performance posts on Facebook, "I wish I could rock this look every day!"

Along with redefining a larger belly as beautiful and revealing one's stomach while dancing, belly dance also helps participants feel better about their bodies because cultural ideals of attractiveness around the globe vary. Western standards of beauty are not necessarily shared in other parts of the world. The yardstick by which some dancers evaluate their appearance changes when they enter the world of belly dance. Along with adorning their bodies in clothing that borrows elements from non-Western cultures, some seasoned dancers tell stories about voluptuous women in the Middle East being more desirable than their thinner counterparts. Using different cultural lenses through which to judge themselves helps some dancers feel more attractive. "I am a larger woman," Alexandra proclaims. "I have blonde hair and both those things tend to draw Arab men in the audience to extremes of emotion," she explains. "Sometimes I can just walk out on stage and toss my hair over my shoulder, and I can get applause for it. So of course that is very good for my self-esteem," she says even though she does not consider herself the "world's greatest dancer." As we have seen throughout this chapter, Alexandra's experiences illustrate the "looking-glass body." She presents her body (and hair) on stage, she receives affirming applause for her appearance, and she feels good about herself as a result of the positive feedback.

Barbara believes that in Egypt or Lebanon, "the audience starts to swoon over plus size dancers." At one point, she considered herself a larger dancer. Barbara tells me about a performance at which a Middle Eastern gentlemen approached her husband at the time and said "your wife is so fat" as he grinned. Not fully understanding cultural differences, Barbara's husband calmly replied, "Yeah OK. The guy clearly thought it was a compliment, and that it was a *big* compliment!" Barbara exclaims.

Exercising, gaining confidence, meeting the challenge of moving the body in new ways, and redefining physical beauty are fairly uncontested bodily norms inside belly dance circles. However, while some internal subcultural messages achieve a relatively high level of agreement among members, others spark more debate. The extent to which the dance is viewed as sexual is one of the most prominent contested beliefs among belly dancers.

The contested belly dancing sexual body

Because a dancing body is on display for people to gaze upon, it is considered to represent both power and sexuality (Albright 1997). Much like sexual tensions in tango (Tobin 1998), the sexual aspects of belly dance are highly contested. However, while sexuality is controversial among female dancers, it is less problematic among the men. Rather than emphasizing sexuality, many of the men with whom I spoke attempted to downplay any sexual aspects of belly dance.

Henry distinguishes between sexuality and sensuality in belly dance. "Belly dance by its very nature is sensual, but it's not sexual," Henry tells me. Rather than being "blatant and obvious," Henry suggests sensuality in belly dance is more suggestive. "There might be a little sensuality to it because of the nature of the movements, but it's not sexual at all say compared to a burlesque show where someone can get very overt and sexual in their act. I try to keep it as vaguely sexual, whereas other female dancers can get away with a little more sexual in their dancing," he tells me. Henry's comments suggest that it is more problematic for him to stress sexuality in his dance compared to his female counterparts. Rather than sexuality, Henry focuses more on entertainment. Henry strives to showcase "happy and exuberant." I wonder how he projects these traits. It's in the "facial expressions and arm movements," Henry explains. Henry tries to project outward toward the audience rather than focusing on himself partly to control any sexuality that may come through in his dance.

In fact, Henry expresses concern that a top he wore for a previous performance was too "risqué." He was so concerned that his shirt was too inappropriately sexual that he did not want me to use any pictures from his performance in this book. The top is a mesh material that is more sheer than what he typically wears. Henry's nipples are visible through the thin covering and "I felt very self-conscious about that. I was hoping with the light it wouldn't be visible," he tells me. Henry feels more comfortable when he is "covered up." "I never perform topless ... So I felt last night's costume was a bit on the more risqué side." Like Henry's actions, men are often encouraged to monitor their sexual expressions (Kimmel 2008).

Male dancers most likely downplay sexuality in their dance because they are aware of and highly sensitive to how their presence affects female dancers. Many of the men do not want to make the women uncomfortable, which may happen if they were overtly sexual. "One of the things I try to do is to let women know I'm a peer, I'm not there to hit on them," Henry tells me. Although he has dated belly dancers who live hundreds of miles away from him, Henry has never dated a dancer inside his immediate belly dance community. He wants his fellow dancers know that "I'm there because I want to dance," Henry explains.

Like Henry, Kevin is keenly aware of how his presence could affect the women in his dance class. His classes are structured in twelve-week segments. Every three months, a new set of people join the classes. He tells me:

> You've got to let that group get used to you. It helps to reassure them that you aren't there to hit on them ... I do kind of wonder what thoughts are going through the heads of these girls. Is this guy gay? Is he a cross dresser? Is he here to hit on us? It takes them a while to get used to me and realize I am perfectly safe and not going to do anything.

"Is there anything you do to help the women feel like you aren't a threat?" I inquire. Much like Henry who does not date inside his immediate belly dance community, Kevin "does not hit on" the women in his classes. "In general, I keep to myself ... I just come there, I dance and occasionally chat with a few of my friends, and that's about it," Kevin explains. Kevin and Henry illustrate that male dancers downplay their sexuality partially out of concern for how they will be perceived by the female dancers, and this containing of sexuality is highly agreed upon among male dancers.

However, sexuality among the women belly dancers is subject to great controversy. On one hand, many female dancers use belly dance to help them feel sexy. "I feel pretty and sometimes sexy, which is something when you are my age and my size," Dena, in her fifties, comments. As a larger than average sized woman, she continues, "It's really something to feel sexy, because it's not what you see on TV as sexy," Dena says to me, reiterating my earlier discussion of belly dance welcoming, and defining as beautiful, bodies of various shapes, sizes, and ages.

When Sydney first got involved in belly dance, she chose the persona of a belly dancer over another period character for an event she attended. "What did you like about the idea of belly dance?" I ask her. Sydney replies, "In my mind it was that James Bond type of sexy thing. That sexy woman, and I was like, 'OOO.' I wanted people to be like, 'Look at her! She's amazing!'" Sydney was shown a picture of the other period character she had the option to portray and she was reminded of wearing maternity outfits. With several children, Sydney says, "I don't need any more of those clothes."

Some dancers acknowledge that audience members gaze upon their bodies and offer positive feedback about a dancer's beauty and/or the quality of her dance. Many female dancers are unapologetic that they enjoy that attention and validation. It boosts their self-confidence and helps them feel good about their bodies and appearance. "Is belly dance sexual or sensual for you?" I ask Alexandra. "Oh yes! I don't know why that is supposed to be a bad thing," she quickly responds. "Some people are very adamant that 'no, belly dance is not something sexual. It's about art.' Well, what is wrong with it being about sex?" Alexandra thinks that belly dance has a sexual component to it, but she realizes that her position may not be a popular one. "I try not to say that too loud because there would be even more tension in the belly dance community than there needs to be. But some people, maybe sometimes the loudest people, are the ones that say 'it's not about sex or pleasing men,'" she continues. Alexandra admits that "I kind of like it when a dozen men shout I love you." "Am I supposed to pretend like I don't enjoy that?" she rhetorically asks while acknowledging the internal debates within belly dance circles.

I spend a Saturday afternoon at a belly dance event with workshops and an evening show. I run into an old friend with whom I danced many years prior. It has been awhile since we have seen each other, so I ask, "What have you been up?" "I've gotten more into burlesque dancing," my friend quietly responds. She reaches into her shoulder bag and removes a flyer for an upcoming burlesque show. "I didn't think they would want me to put these flyers on the table," my friend explains. She did not feel that her burlesque advertisements would be welcomed next to belly dance related materials given the prevailing opinion that belly dance should remain separate from (presumably sexualized) burlesque acts. Swimmers do not acknowledge their state of "near nakedness" because doing so would disrupt the agreed upon meaning of the activity (Scott 2009). Likewise, to publicly acknowledge any sexual aspect of belly dance may disturb the "polite fiction" (Burns 1992) that there is nothing at all sexual about belly dance.

Similar to Henry's comments, one way many female dancers navigate the contested nature of sexuality is to draw strong distinctions between sexuality and sensuality. Rather than seeing themselves as objects of someone else's pleasure, some dancers cast themselves as subjects who dance in ways that they find sensual. "It's not the hips or the breasts, but it's the bare belly that makes it so feminine. It's very sensual," Peg explains. She says that belly dance "can be sensual without being sexual." She suggests that "sensuality is an attitude . . . anything sexual is the promise of something more." "Sensuality incorporates the five senses. The senses are inflamed," Peg states. Peg engages in role-distance by symbolically distinguishing between sensuality and sexuality. Role-distance is a wedge between an individual and some aspect of a role they play with which they do not want to identify (Goffman 1961). There is a quiet acknowledgment that many participants like belly dance because it helps them feel sexy or sensual. At the same time, there is a quick assertion that it is an artful or otherwise more wholesome kind of sensuality that is different to other kinds of dance.

Similarly, Ophelia feels "sexy when she dances," but suggests that belly dance is "sexual in a good way." "Some people think it's a sexual dance, and it's not. Part of it is, but not the whole part. Not in a vulgar way," Ophelia says. "How is it sexual in a good way?" I ask. "I guess as a woman for yourself, discovering how your body moves. I didn't know my hips moved that way! It doesn't matter what size you are, whenever you can do something that makes you feel good," Ophelia remarks. "It is becoming myself, a woman, more in tuned with my body as a belly dancer," she continues. "I think we are taught to shove that down and not let that be a part of it, but I don't think it's a bold sexuality," she comments.

Peg, Ophelia, and Alexandra highlight the ambivalent relationship that some dancers have toward sexuality and belly dance. On one hand, many dancers appreciate how belly dance helps them feel sexy and desirable. At the same time, they symbolically distinguish the sexuality they see in belly dance as different and not as potentially problematic as the sexuality that may be associated with other dance forms. To acknowledge that belly dance is at least partly sexual might imply that it is similar to erotic dancing. Furthermore, it touches on larger cultural apprehension about female sexuality.

Subcultures are not isolated from their surrounding culture. Although subcultures have their internal norms and values, these ideals are influenced by the larger culture in which it is situated. In the United States, there is much ambivalence surrounding sexuality (Barkan 2004), and female sexuality has long been considered suspect and deviant. Women have been reprimanded for wearing indecent clothing, held responsible for a man's arousal, and had their sexual desire labeled an illness (D'Emilio and Freedman 1997; Tolman 2002). Excessive female sexual desire is frowned upon, and women are expected to have smaller sexual appetites compared to men (D'Emilio and Freedman 1997; Salutin 1971). Therefore, when women behave sexually, it is assumed they do so for other people (Tolman 2002). At the same time, women are told they need protection from men who are encouraged to have a strong sexual desire. Women are expected to simultaneously be attractive to and sheltered from men (Bartky 1990). Perhaps it is understanding these mixed messages that are sent to women that results in male dancers downplaying sexuality and attempting to appear non-threatening toward female dancers.

As a result of these mixed cultural messages, women may fear their own sexuality. It is difficult for them to think of themselves as sexual beings on their own terms with the right to sexual pleasure and sexual safety (Tolman 2002). They can feel guilty, uneasy with their femaleness, and experience bodily shame (Bordo 2003). In this way, larger cultural ideas about (particularly female) sexuality infiltrate belly dance and are expressed in the highly controversial ways that dancers talk about sexuality within the dance. Along with sexuality, despite the fact that internal messages are fairly consistent in regards to body acceptance, (particularly female) belly dancers are not immune to Western cultural norms regarding how a female body should appear.

Cultural ideals contaminate body positivity

We learn to see ourselves and our bodies through interactions and the messages we receive from the media, our family, our co-workers, and our peers (Clarke 2011; Clarke and Griffin 2007, 2008). Women are taught that thinner is better than heavier, and toned and healthy is better than flabby and unhealthy. At the same time, women are expected to maintain a curvaceous and "feminine" appearance (Bordo 2003; Grogan 2008). The thin body is the only type deemed socially acceptable and has become a core measure of a woman's femininity (Connell 2002; Hesse-Biber 2006; Murray 2004). Women are typically valued to the degree that they meet these cultural ideals and receive rewards and punishments based on how their bodies measure up to these norms (Bordo 2003; Hesse-Biber 2006; Jeffreys 2005; Wolf 1990). However, cultural standards for feminine beauty are so narrow that, by some estimates, less than 10 percent of the female population can live up to these ideals (Kilbourne 1994).

Failing to adhere to cultural norms can leave women feeling unhappy with their appearance (Bordo 2003; Clarke 2011; Fredrickson and Roberts 1997; Griffith 2004; Grogan 2008; Striegel-Moore and Franko 2002; Weinberg and Williams 2010). In fact, women's dissatisfaction with their bodies is so pervasive that Bordo (2003:186) argues that focusing on weight is "one of the most powerful normalizing mechanisms of our century" which sustains self-monitoring and disciplining bodily practices. Although this pattern is consistent across all groups of women, body dissatisfaction is particularly tied to women in higher socio-economic groups and women with higher levels of education (Abell and Richards 1996; McLauren and Kuh 2004). Interestingly, the women in this study are well educated with the vast majority finishing college and almost one-third possessing a graduate or professional degree. Because our bodies and selves are linked, we judge ourselves poorly when our bodies are stigmatized (Goffman 1963).

Norms about the way a woman's body should look vary by audience and location. Many women find acceptance of body and age diversity within their local belly dance communities. However, when dancers perform at regional or national belly dance events or in front of a general audience at restaurants, clubs, and festivals, there is more pressure to adhere to cultural norms regarding physical attractiveness. In this way, the mirror that reflects an image back to the dancer is altered. Thus, a dancer's view of herself can change.

Earlier, I discussed an interaction during which a Middle Eastern man complimented Barbara's husband for being married to a "fat" woman. Although Barbara understands that this man's affirmation was rooted in his culture's definition of feminine beauty, she spent over a year losing a great deal of weight. Barbara partly felt she would be hired to teach more workshops throughout the United States if she was thinner. About difficulties she experiences in belly dance, Barbara begins by saying, "It has been recently about how I need to look." She continues, "It wasn't as much of a problem before, but as I'm getting more advanced and well known, [her body] has been an interesting challenge. I just have some pressure to shed some pounds, both from me and from the community in general." Many dancers who are well known for the style of dance that Barbara performs are very petite women (see Figure 3.1). "I think it's harder to make it as a bigger sized lady," Barbara confides. Barbara has a belly dance friend whom she considers very talented, but is larger than average workshop instructors. She believes they are both skilled enough to lead regional or national workshops, "but it's very hard for us to get them," Barbara explains. "I feel like it's harder than someone who is thinner," she continues. She also feels her costumes highlight her "bulges," which makes her feel uneasy. So losing the weight is "for my self-confidence and for getting those workshop

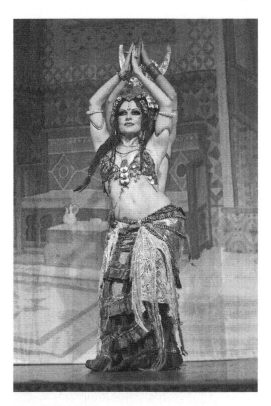

Figure 3.1 Tribal fusion dancer

Photo credit: Carrie Meyer/The Dancers Eye.

opportunities and getting more recognition for being thinner." Professional dancers are pressured to maintain certain weights and a desirable appearance. There is little bodily variation in some professional dance companies and many dance cultures include unhealthy bodily behaviors, such as extreme dieting and exercise, with the goal of achieving and maintaining a culturally accepted look (Albright 1997). In Barbara's case, she has dieted off and on over the years. Although her weight has fluctuated, she remains thinner than when she started and she is now being hired to teach workshops in her region.

At the local level, belly dance invites one set of subjective views, while regional or national audiences may offer different subjective views. Belly dancers manage multiple subjective views and reflect on their bodies differently using whatever mirror is most relevant or applicable at that moment. Lana has earned her living through belly dance for many years. Many of the women with whom Lana used to work "got boob jobs and face lifts and this was nipped and tucked, and years later something else nipped and tucked," she tells me. "Was that because they were performing in a commercial setting?" I wonder about the well-known theme park that attracted visitors across the country at which Lana used to dance regularly. "I think they felt that way," Lana replies. Although she did not participate in body modification to the extent of some of her fellow dancers, "I do believe in costuming enhancement," she admits.

Over the "thousands" of belly grams (performances at private events) that Lana has performed, "it isn't unusual for someone to ask 'what do you look like? How old are you? Are you fat?'" She tells me. "I always lied about my age because I look younger," she continues. Lana believes passing for someone who is thirty-five is acceptable to a potential client, "but forty-five is not going to be OK with them because they are looking at their forty-five-year-old wife or next door neighbor . . . and you aren't going to get that job," Lana explains. "They want a certain look, and they don't care that much if you can dance or not." "I've even had them say, 'do you have big boobs? We want someone with big boobs,'" Lana continues. She would respond, "I sure do!" "We all pad our bras," she tells me. "You want to round out the figure. It's an aesthetic. You are supposed to have big boobs and big hips. You want to shoot for the hourglass figure. It's just like makeup," she explains. In these ways, Lana and other dancers engage in what Meltzer (2003) identifies as "self-enhancement fabrications," such as embellishing a job application or resume and using various cosmetic tools to create a different and more desirable appearance.

"I don't have the best body image," Taylor tells me. "I would never expose my abdomen simply because it would make me feel so self-conscious while I was dancing." She frequently wears leotards or full-length dresses when she dances (see Figure 3.2). "I just don't reveal my stomach. One year, I bought a leotard with a sheer middle. I was uncomfortable the entire time I had it on. I would rather be thinner. I had been, and I know I could be," Taylor explains. Vannini and Waskul (2006:189) define body ekstasis as "the qualitative evaluation of the aesthetic potential of one's body" as judged against other bodies and one's potential. In some cases, we become dissatisfied with our bodies when we evaluate them against other bodies and how we think our bodies could look. Taylor's comments illustrate her value judgment of her body based on the fact that she believes it's possible for her to have a smaller frame.

Furthermore, Taylor tells me, "I am firmly in the camp that says no one wants to see my middle. At my age, I think it's inappropriate. Somehow, the idea of [an older] woman parading around with a lot of skin showing is kind of icky." Taylor comments on societal expectations regarding dress when she says, "I think there is appropriate wear for every age group, and I think I'm in the no bare midriff, no bikinis, no short shorts, no boob display age group, and that suits me just fine." Although she opts for costumes that fully cover her arms, chest, and midriff, Taylor believes that "those choices seem to neither lessen

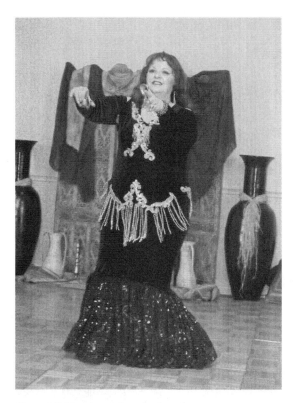

Figure 3.2 Dancer performing in a dress
Photo credit: Courtesy of Lynn Ciurej.

my enjoyment in doing this dance nor the audiences' enjoyment in watching." In fact, she continues to receive many compliments and praise of her dancing. Although many participants view belly dance as a safe site for body diversity, at the same time, several dancers feel apprehensive about displaying their bodies that do not conform to stereotypical notions of Western beauty. Unlike Barbara who has lost a great deal of weight and Lana who pads her bra, Taylor opts to more fully cover her body. Rather than altering her body to conform to Western ideas of beauty, she chooses to conceal aspects of her body that she believes some members of the general public may find unappealing.

I rarely post pictures of myself in a belly dance costume on the Internet partly because I do not normally find belly dance costumes to be flattering on me. However, I posted a picture on my Facebook page from a performance at a renaissance festival (see Figure 3.3). Despite having a different body type than professional, nationally well-known belly dancers (see Figures 3.1 and 3.4), I like the way I look in this photograph. Although I am happy with my appearance in

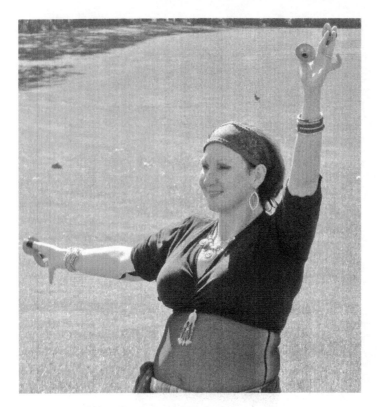

Figure 3.3 Rachel performing at a festival

Photo credit: Scott A. Desmond.

this picture, the reader will notice the sheer black stocking that I have over my middle, which functions to at least partly cover my stomach.

While some dancers love playing "dress up," and enjoy the costumes, other dancers have ambivalent feelings toward the amount of skin that is exposed in some belly dance attire. One of the reasons why I am less comfortable in belly dance clothing is because I, like Taylor and some other dancers, am not comfortable exposing my belly. Dancers like myself and Taylor are affected by traditional Western notions of beauty. Some dancers feel their bellies are larger than what Western cultural standards of beauty dictate, so they wear various coverings. In fact, I never show my bare stomach during my dance classes, informal gatherings, rehearsals, or performances. Frankly, I am most exposed when I wear a sheer covering over my midriff, and I only typically wear a sheer covering as dictated by my troupe's costuming preferences for any given performance. When I have an option, I generally choose the black sheer stocking or a black lace covering.

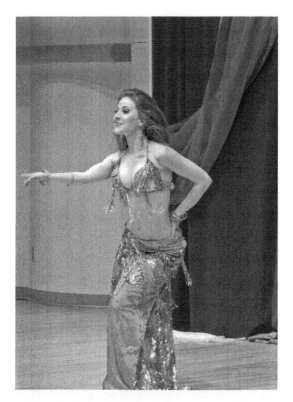

Figure 3.4 Cabaret style belly dance superstar

Belly dance costumes help women do femininity by assisting some participants in creating a culturally accepted appearance rooted in stereotypical notions of feminine beauty. Even when our stomachs are larger than cultural values of thinness may dictate, other aspects of costuming, such as skirts, heavy makeup, and neatly styled hair can help women more closely approximate typical notions of attractiveness. When one aspect of traditional feminine beauty is not met (thinness), an overall pleasing look is achieved by the successful incorporation of other typical feminine tools, such as gender-specific dress, makeup, accessories, jewelry, and hairstyles.

In 2013, my husband, Scott, and I attend a Bellydance Superstar show called *Club Bellydance*. The Bellydance Superstars is a professional international group that performs various belly dance shows all over the world. *Club Bellydance* begins with performances by several local belly dancers from the surrounding areas. After several acts, there is an intermission and the remaining performances are given by a few members of the Bellydance Superstars. Scott and I thoroughly enjoy both segments of the show. As we discuss the various acts, Scott remarks that he does not see much difference between the quality of the dancing or the entertainment value in the two sections. Scott may not have the keenest eye for belly dance technique, performance, or stage presence. But he does make one very interesting observation: the local dancers represent a range of ages, heights, and body shapes while the Bellydance Superstar performers fit a narrower definition of attractiveness that closely mirrors Western cultural ideals (in fact the vast majority of Bellydance Superstars are under the age of forty). All of the Bellydance Superstars dancers were also Caucasian (see Figure 3.4). They displayed long hair (or long hair pinned up with hair ornaments as dictated by the style of dance they performed). Scott's observation about the appearance of the local dancers and that of the Bellydance Superstars impressed upon me the challenge of meeting cultural standards of beauty when dancers want to perform nationally and attempt to make a living at belly dance.

Given that dance is first and foremost a bodily practice, messages about the body are constantly disseminated within belly dance communities. Much of this bodily rhetoric is uncontested, particularly those ideas that align fairly easily with predominant cultural ideals. Our society tells us that it is "good" to engage in health-enhancing bodily practices. When dancers physically cannot participate in or do not enjoy traditional forms of exercise, they use belly dance as a way to participate in "healthism," while doing so in unique ways. The unusual ways of moving the body provide a challenge that allows many dancers to feel a sense of physical accomplishment, when they otherwise may not be able to do so.

At the same time, those areas of contention within belly dance subvert popular notions about the female body and sexuality. Body image is a tricky issue within belly dance. Inside their classrooms, immediate geographical areas, and among belly dance audiences, gazing upon a variety of ages and body sizes helps women and men who do not conform to stereotypical notions of attractiveness feel better about their own appearance. At the same time, when their bodies are displayed for a broader audience who arguably operate more from traditional Western norms of beauty, dancers navigate these competing values, but do so in different ways. Some dancers alter their bodies (or at least their body's appearance) in ways that closer conform to these traditional ideals, while others cover their bodies so as to not "offend" Western audiences.

Whereas issues surrounding body image require reconciling internal belly dance community norms with external cultural ideals regarding beauty, debates about sexuality mostly occur inside the world of belly dance. However, like issues of body image, perhaps sexuality in belly dance may be so contested because of the larger cultural ambivalence regarding (primarily female) sexuality. Therefore, to some degree, contested and uncontested messages internal to belly dance hinge on, or at least are influenced by, the extent to which they align with outside cultural values.

Chapter 4

Friendship and community

They all seem to be sisterly toward each other. When we are together we all just help each other however we can, and I really enjoy that.

(Elisa, 50s, four years in belly dance)

In some ways, arriving at this hafla is standard for me. I attended this gathering the previous summer, so I am somewhat familiar with the location, set up, people, and the program for the evening. It is a fairly popular and well-attended event that draws belly dancers from across the region. During the day, multiple instructors from all over the United States offer specialized workshops ranging from makeup artistry, costuming, and layering belly dance movements, to perfecting arm positions. In the evening, the instructors of these workshops and other local dancers perform in an evening show. Vendors display costume pieces, jewelry, books, and DVDs on tables in the common purpose room. This year's event is particularly meaningful. The emcee stands in front of the performance area facing the sea of chairs and audience members. She announces that half of the proceeds from the event will be donated to another dancer to help cover expenses for a recently diagnosed health condition that requires a very expensive medical procedure. Along with the sales from vending and admission tickets, collections from a donation box will be given to the dancer. She talks fondly about her dance sister, expresses sincere gratitude for the money that has already come in, and kindly encourages us to continue giving and/or purchase items from the vendors.

One Friday evening, one of my dance sisters and I drive to a drum circle. After about a thirty-minute commute we arrive at the warehouse-type building and my dance sister who is driving parks her van. We sit for a few minutes while she punches buttons on her cell phone. I silently wonder what she is doing. "Why aren't we going inside?" I think to myself. Maybe my fellow dancer caught on to my confusion as to why we were sitting in her parked van at our destination. She explains that she is texting with a mutual dance friend of ours who is in the process of purchasing a car. My dance sister is married to someone who works in the automobile industry. She and her husband have provided our mutual friend with car advice over the years, so our mutual friend turned to her for some assistance with her new car purchase. Although

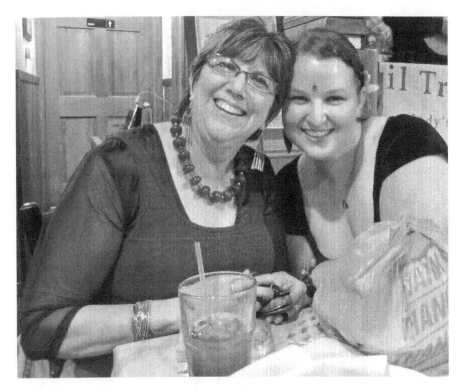

Figure 4.1 Troupe sisters meet at a restaurant to dance to some local music

some dancers receive a great deal of support when they or someone close to them is faced with serious health diagnoses, participants also help each other with more mundane situations in everyday life. Dancers offer advice, assistance, and job leads to one another.

Many women develop friendships in belly dance, and they think about these relationships as a "sisterhood" (Moe 2012, 2014). In this chapter, I investigate how friendships within belly dance are formed and maintained (see Figure 4.1). For many female swimmers, the swimming pool is a venue for socializing and building friendships (Scott 2010). Belly dance, like swimming, is another site to "do friendship." In fact, some participants find stronger friendships within belly dance than any other place in their life. For these participants, belly dance speaks to an "impulse to sociability" (Simmel 1949:254). In other words, participants derive satisfaction from an activity simply by associating with other people. Interacting with others can create feelings of togetherness (Simmel 1949). Within subcultures, friendship is partially accomplished through participants spending a great deal of time together (Wilkins 2008). Belly dancers see each other on a regular basis in weekly classes, rehearsals, workshops, and haflas.

Doing friendship

Female friendships offer a wide range of benefits, including a positive effect on their well-being, feelings of connection, self-esteem, happiness, increased life expectancy, and a buffer against stress and anxiety (Aleman 2010; Comas-Diaz and Weiner 2013; Felder 2006; Knickmeyer *et al.* 2002; O'Conner 1992). These relationships offer women comfort, security, relaxation, and emotional support (Aries and Johnson 1983; Bernard 1981; Comas-Diaz and Weiner 2013). Belly dancers "do friendship" in a variety of ways and benefit from these relationships.

"It's almost like group therapy"

Talking, emotional sharing, and discussing personal problems with their same-sex friends is a crucial component for maintaining and constructing women's friendships (Coates 1996). In fact, Green (1998) argues that women's talk is the most satisfying aspect of participating in leisure. In her twenties, Candie had some particularly challenging family health issues. Although she receives solace from other outlets, the encouragement is "not as much as [what she finds in] belly dance." Candie likens belly dance to "an open forum for women to discuss issues." When she is in belly dance classes or instructional dance seminars, the attendees "always end up talking about so much more than just dance," Candie tells me. She and the women in her classes "talk about life and stress. It's almost like group therapy," Candie says. "You have this open and unconditional love from these other women, and I think you don't always get that in different aspects of society. Girls that I don't dance with send me supportive emails on a regular basis," Candie explains. "My mom has [cancer]. It's crazy just the love and support I have got from people that I haven't talked to in such a long time . . . everybody just kind of stepped up to the plate. I don't see that in some of the other facets of my life."

"They were so helpful through difficult times of finding myself again," Lilly says about the friendships she formed with some of her troupe sisters. They "helped me feel better about myself again," Lilly fondly remembers. Lilly recalls when she was working on a graduate degree while in a long-distance relationship. Her boyfriend confessed to cheating on her with several women. In addition, "I found out he is a pathological liar," and he was involved in various illegal activities. Needless to say, Lilly was devastated. "This person wasn't the person I thought he was. All these people knew but never told me," she sadly remembers. Lilly did not have many friends in her academic program because she traveled out of town quite a bit on the weekends to see her boyfriend. "I wasn't feeling too good about myself. I just didn't trust people,"

Lilly recalls. Although Lilly had difficulty depending on people in general, "I started making friends in belly dancing. I had these female friends . . . we could talk about our crises and everyone had something in their past, and we celebrated the good things in each other." For dancers such as Candie and Lilly, belly dance provides an important setting in which participants can talk with other women about their personal lives. In these cases, the conversations center on providing support for each other. Receiving support, encouragement, and advice contributes to building friendships.

"It helps me be a little more outgoing"

Scott (2005) argues that many people who are shy recognize that being shy is potentially a "discreditable" flaw. In other words, if other people realize a person is shy, they may view the person as awkward and avoid him or her. As a result, the shy person may have fewer social ties, receive less social support, and feel marginalized. Wanting to avoid negative consequences, some people who are shy seek out ways to minimize their shyness. Participants who think of themselves as shy, misfits, or lonely discover a sense of belonging in dance (Shay 2008). Belly dance helps some participants to be more social because it helps them become less shy. Being more outgoing and social is conducive to building both friendships and community.

Larry appreciates one of his instructors who helps her students "break out of that shell" and "get out there more." "Can you describe the shell for me?" I inquire. "I have always been a very shy person," Larry replies. When he was little, Larry would hide behind his mother whenever people approached him. "So I have always just been very shy, and even growing up I wasn't ever part of a particular circle. I tried to avoid the spotlight as much as possible. I was just kind of staying in the background. [Belly dance] is kind of helping me get out there and be a little bit more outgoing with people and talking to them more," Larry says. Scott (2005) argues that shyness can intersect with other characteristics, such as gender. Some of Scott's (2005) participants suggested that shyness is more socially acceptable for women, who are "allowed" to be more quiet and reserved, compared to men who are expected to have a more commanding presence and be in charge (Scott 2005). Therefore, shyness is more challenging for men like Larry to navigate as it violates norms of masculinity more so than expectations of femininity. As a result, men especially may appreciate activities that help them overcome shyness.

Like Larry, Abigail considers herself shy. She intentionally constructs her belly dance persona to be more social than how she regularly sees herself. Abigail views belly dance performing as "acting a little bit more than being myself." "It sounds like it's different than what you would be outside of dancing," I comment. "Yeah, I think it helps me be a little more outgoing, and that can be good thing," Abigail replies.

For Abigail, Larry, and some other dancers, belly dance helps them contend with their shyness. Scott (2005) suggests that along with worrying about embarrassing oneself, shyness also results from concerns regarding consequences that may stem from not living up to others' expectations. Belly dance is an outlet that helps people develop a feeling of confidence so they are less concerned about any "performance" falling short of others' expectations. Scott (2005) identifies shyness as occupying an awkward position of not being completely absent from a situation, but not completely immersed in it. Especially when belly dancers perform in any kind of setting, shyness is not an option. A dancer is displayed on a literal stage. She or he does not have the option to hide in a corner. Situations with some structure, rules, and scripted behavior can help people momentarily overcome their shyness (Scott 2005) and that is precisely what some people find within belly dance. A belly dance performance, especially a choreographed one, offers a set of formal rules about when to be on stage, how long to be on stage, and what movements to perform while on stage. This predetermined structure no doubt facilitates taking a break from shyness. Like other shy individuals (Scott 2005), belly dancers play a fairly defined role within a safe and temporary space. Under these scripted and pre-set conditions of performing, the uncertainty over how to act is removed. Knowing what to expect in a given situation, such as the steps in a dance and the music, helps dancers relax.

"What do you think helps you maintain your relationship with dancers outside of the dance?" I ask Dena. "I am social and always have been," Dena replies. Although she considers herself social, as a self-identified introvert, Dena explains, "being social is a choice for me, and it often takes some psyching myself out to accomplish it." "Being social in dance circles is much easier than being social in everyday situations," Dena tells me. "In dance groups, you already have a shared passion about which to talk and connect. In everyday situations, you are always looking for that something on which you can connect. We keep our introverted selves well hidden," Dena continues. Because of the commonality of the dance, Dena "finds it pretty easy to socialize and not feel stressed in dance situations." In addition to the stage offering a formal structure guiding participants on how to act, having belly dance as a common activity provides participants with a pre-existing topic of conversation, which eases their interactions.

The summer time is ripe with festivals and outdoor public gatherings. One unseasonably cool summer evening, I attend a street festival in a town at which some belly dancers perform. During a break between their acts, a few of the dancers order dinner at a local restaurant. I hang out with them while they wait for their food. The previous day, I had asked members of this group about their friendships with belly dancers. Without my prompt, a few of the dancers begin talking about this question I posed the day earlier. "That's because 95 per cent of us are introverts," one of the dancers announces while they are sitting around the table waiting for their food to arrive. Her comments mirror Dena's sentiments. "Put me in a costume, and I can dance on stage. But the costume is a completely different persona," she continues. One of the other dancers remarked how she sits at a desk in the back of the room at her day job and listens to music in relative solitude. For dancers like the few in this group, belly dance helps them be more extroverted and spend time with other people within the context of the dance. In Chapter 2, I suggested that putting on a belly dance costume can act as a "second skin" in that what we wear penetrates us and becomes a little of who we are (Goffman 1974). Putting on a costume also helps some dancers become more extroverted and social.

Over the years, Dena has watched some of her students transform when they put on belly dance costumes. "I think of them as the superheroes of belly dance – for how well they are disguised in their everyday looks," Dena tells me about a few of her former students. "I think when they dance, they stand taller, hold themselves more confidently, etc. They do more with hair and makeup, so they look different than in everyday life," Dena explains. She continues to illustrate her analogy when she says, "all superheroes have a costume that supposedly makes them unidentifiable when they are just their everyday personas." In fact, Dena used to refer to a dancer friend of hers as the "Superman of belly dance." "Seen without the makeup and costuming, she was just this everyday person with bowl cut hair and dark rimmed glasses. But then she steps on the stage in makeup, no glasses, and a fancy costume and va-va-voom!" Dena exclaims. "Fantasy – part of why we all love playing dress-up in belly dance." Dena astutely describes how getting dressed in belly dance costumes can alter not only one's appearance, but a dancer's personality. Inside the pool, the identity of the swimmer becomes a master status where all other identities are placed on the back burner (Scott 2010). Much like swimmers who change into swim suits, enter a pool, and immerse themselves in swimming (Scott 2010), when belly dancers put on a costume, they step into a world beyond their ordinary existence and leave their other identities behind.

"I'm more extroverted when I'm on stage," Henry tells me. As a self-proclaimed introvert, "being in public is exhausting" to Henry. If Henry does something in public, he needs to sit by himself for about an hour to "re-center." But, "once I put on my costume, I'm a different person. It's that ritual of putting on a costume that aspects of my personality change. I become much more outgoing because that is what is necessary to be the performer," Henry explains. Engaging in a very public activity during which one typically receives much support and affirmation facilitates participants becoming more social.

Belly dance provides a script that guides dancers on how they perform and interact with other dancers and audience members. When they follow the guidelines, dancers who consider themselves "shy" or "introverted" play a more social and extroverted role. Being more social increases interactions with other people and aids in the building of friendships. Furthermore, regular interaction with the same small group of people over years provides opportunities to become more comfortable with and get to know group members better, which enhances the building of friendships. Finally, focusing on an activity that people can enjoy together and doesn't require a lot of talking can help some introverts feel connected to other dancers.

"People are going to be cheering for you"

Norms that govern belly dance shows dictate that audiences make noise during the various acts to encourage the performers. The expectations of audiences at belly dance displays differ from the norm to sit quietly that operates at other artistic performances. Emcees at many belly dance events teach the audience about "proper" etiquette before a show begins. In this sense, the emcee "defines the situation" (Thomas and Thomas 1928) as an audience participation and interactive performance. In addition to zaghareet, which I described earlier, audiences may yell "yallah," which loosely translated means, "let's go." It is also acceptable to "yip" or call out "aiwa" (pronounced like Iowa, but replace the "i" with an "a" sound, which is slang for "yes"). I have also observed hissing and meow sounds during performances featuring slow movements. This active involvement from the audience is interpreted by a performer as enjoying the show, whereas silence is sometimes interpreted as boredom.

Maggie likes performing particularly for other belly dancers. "The belly dance audience is by far the best," Maggie tells me, and adds, "It doesn't matter if you are choking up there or if you are really doing good, people are going to be cheering for you." Dancers such as Maggie appreciate positive feedback they receive from audiences. When some belly dancers receive support and praise during performances, they feel more secure in their ability and perhaps offer an even better show. In this sense, the relationship between the performer and the audience is circular and each relies on the other for the best experience.

Maggie's experiences are not unlike concerts or sporting events where fans cheer on players or groupies scream and dance along to music. Her experiences are also similar to the interaction between teacher and student in an academic classroom in that the quality of a class session often depends on the participation and attentiveness of the students. Furthermore, the relationship between belly dancer and audience member mirrors the connection between preacher and congregation member in religious groups that rely on interaction for a meaningful worship service. Positive feedback from congregations can boost preachers' confidence and help them offer a better worship experience. However, it can be challenging for a preacher to fulfill his or her duties if the congregation is nonresponsive (Nelson 1996). Likewise, it can be difficult for belly dancers to perform for audiences that appear to lack enthusiasm. Because norms internal to belly dance communities call for dancers to support one another and to verbally show their appreciation during performances, performers are likely to feel supported and encouraged, which helps them feel connected to their fellow dancers. Feeling close to other dancers leads to building friendships with them.

"They are always going to be accepting"

Many belly dance communities emphasize their acceptance of diversity. Similar to feeling supported, many dancers feel accepted in belly dance. Dena's interactions when she first got involved in belly dance left a lasting impression on her. Given that she has been dancing for over thirty years, Dena, now in her fifties, still recalls the significance of finding acceptance in belly dance. "It was wonderful," Dena remembers. She immediately felt like she belonged with the other dancers. Along with seeing a range of body types that I discussed in the previous chapter, Dena says, "You could dance even if you weren't that great a dancer. There was a feeling of acceptance that you didn't have to be a star to be able to dance for people." This feeling of affirmation and belonging had such a powerful effect on her that Dena "loved it immediately. I was sunk." We join groups partly for self-enhancement or to seek positive information about ourselves. Group membership strengthens our feelings of belonging and can contribute positively to one's self-esteem. Feeling that others value us provides us with a sense of security and meaning (Burke and Stets 2009).

Like Dena, Larissa believes "You are always going to be beautiful to belly dancers, and they are always going to be accepting." "They'll take anybody in . . . It doesn't matter who you are," Larissa says. Larissa finds a lot of tolerance in belly dance. "You bring somebody new, and they are like 'let's go do this.'" Larissa surmises that she has stayed with belly dance for as long as she has (a little less than a year) because "Everybody just goes together." No doubt it is easier to build friendships with people when we feel comfortable and accepted by them.

Interestingly, when Larissa behaved in a way that her teacher felt was not accepting of other dancers, she was reprimanded. In her study of wannabes, Goths, and Christians, Wilkins (2008) demonstrates how friendships are maintained partly because group members regulate each other's behavior. Members encourage each other to abide by group norms and intervene when people stray from group norms (Wilkins 2008). Understanding what behaviors are sanctioned and which ones are prohibited provides clues to the norms that operate within any community. Larissa attended a festival at which several dancers performed. About one act, Larissa said, "I could probably learn that dance in a half hour." "Compared to what we had been doing, [the choreography] was very simple. So I just said I could probably learn that quickly," Larissa recalls. In response, Larissa remembers her instructor "yelling" at her: "'Don't say things like that! That is so rude,'" as Larissa imitates her instructor's disapproving voice. Similar to girls who punish someone when they suggest that they are better than other members of their group (Goodwin 2002), Larissa's teacher tried to limit feelings of superiority among her students. One reason why Larissa's teacher may have reprimanded her is that the instructor is focused on maintaining a "team impression" (Goffman 1959). In other words, Larissa's instructor wants her group of dancers to give off a particular favorable impression, i.e. one that is respectful and supportive of other dancers as formal norms within belly dance tend to dictate.

"All of the wonderful people you meet"

Another aspect of belly dance that is conducive to forming friendships is the variety of people that one meets through the activity. Group members rarely interact exclusively with each other. Individuals often maintain acquaintances with people outside their immediate social circle and simultaneously belong to multiple groups (Fine 2012a). Likewise, some dancers have memberships in multiple belly dance groups, and dancers frequently meet other people outside of their group at a variety of belly dance events, such as haflas (see Figure 4.2), workshops, and shows that draw belly dancers from around the state, region, and occasionally, the country. Fine (2012a:168) refers to these connected groups as "interlocking networks" because they are tied together by members who maintain friendships across different groups. These linkages create a more expansive sense of belonging within a broader community (Fine 2012a). Therefore, belly dancers not only feel connected to other participants in their immediate communities, but to members of other groups as well.

When Barbara first got involved in belly dance about seven years ago, she thought people eventually get bored or become tired of the activity. "But I haven't reached that yet, and I sense that I'm in this for the long haul for now," Barbara says. Although Barbara is only in her thirties, she jokes with another dancer that "we will be old hags still teaching." Barbara believes that she will continue dancing for the rest of her life because of "all the wonderful

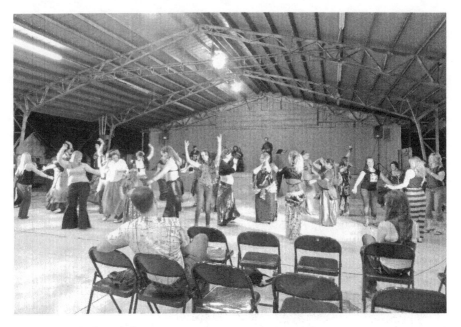

Figure 4.2 Belly dance hafla

people you meet." In fact, Barbara has developed friendships with belly dancers all over the country.

Barbara recently attended a tribal belly dance event that attracts dancers from the region and nationwide. Barbara saw familiar friendly faces, and she enjoyed meeting some new people outside of her immediate dance community. "It's just a marvelous part of the journey to get to know all of those folks," Barbara says. Although her new friends live in another state or in another part of the country, "they feel as much of a part of our tribe as if they were in [Barbara's hometown]. So, we feel like we're in the same community. We've established a bridge between our two communities," Barbara explains.

In addition to the connection between different belly dance groups, dancers are also connected to various drummers and other musicians (see Figures 4.3 and 4.4). Although a drum, or doumbek, is one of the more common instruments used for belly dance music, dancers are also frequently accompanied by musicians playing different instruments, such as the cello or violin, various types of guitars, flutes, clarinets, and the tambourine. There is a relationship that can form between musician and dancer that allows each to play off one another. Some dancers, such as Bobbie, prefer to dance with live music accompaniments because "there is such an intricate relationship with that drummer and the belly dancer," Bobbie explains. "The drummer," she says, is "watching how you dance, and you're listening to how they play." Bobbie suggests that

70

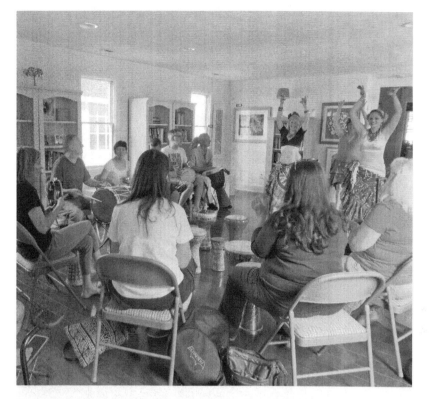

Figure 4.3 Dancers rehearsing during a monthly drum circle

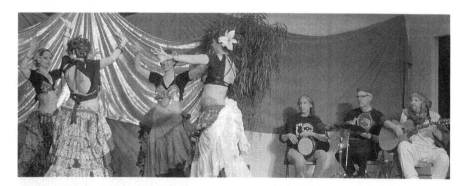

Figure 4.4 American Tribal Style performance accompanied by several musicians

drummers and dancers "feed off of each other" because "it's almost like you are watching them, and they are watching you, and they are adjusting their music to your movements, and you are adjusting your movements to their music, and sometimes that can be a great thing." Dancers and drummers work together to create an aesthetically pleasing visual and audio performance. As such, dancers and musicians within the belly dance community may develop close, professional relationships. Music acts in a way that is different from other non-music activities to structure interactions. It sets a stage and a scene to provide ways of being, behaving, and interacting that can bring people together and foster various kinds of relationships. The fact that people are moving, and moving to music, can help facilitate the friendships they form in a way that is different than if people shared space for a sedentary activity, such as knitting (DeNora 2000).

"They are my kind of girls"

Part of the attractiveness of belly dance for many women is not just making new friends, but forming friendships with other women. Women are given messages that they are "natural enemies" of one another and are taught that it is undesirable to bond with other women (hooks 1984). In fact, some research demonstrates that adolescent girls have negative opinions of other girls, characterizing their female peers as "catty," "backstabbing," and "judgmental" (Crothers et al. 2005). Even as adults, it can be difficult for women to fully support one another because of feeling competitive with other females. As a result, women feel ambivalent about their friendships because they experience love for one another, but they also can feel envious and competitive with their friends (Viorst 1998). Many women who belly dance have experienced these mixed relationships with other women. Belly dance is so meaningful to many of these women precisely because the activity provides an outlet to develop positive female friendships that they may not have typically experienced.

"What do you enjoy about belly dance?" I ask Meredith. "The love I found with other women, my sisters, and the love I have for myself now, which wasn't there before," Meredith replies choking back tears. Belly dance gives Meredith the opportunity "to connect with people socially in ways I couldn't before." Belly dance helps her "appreciate other people and appreciate other woman as well." Meredith believes that "girls can be so mean, which I experienced firsthand, and I'm sure I was mean to plenty of people." Belly dance has helped Meredith value relationships with other women.

One of the reasons why connecting with other women is so meaningful to Meredith is because the attachments that she forms with other dancers are different than her relationships with women outside of belly dance. Meredith observes some of the challenges that girls experience when they are younger when she says, "there are so many different things that happen to girls growing up and they have a hard time dealing with each other and drama." Meredith does not like drama, but she is around a lot of artistic and creative people in her line of work. Even as an adult, she is exposed to a lot of conflict that she calls "overrated." "There's still this love I have for every woman I meet just because she is a woman. That stems from belly dance," Meredith says. "I don't get that anywhere else, especially at [her job]. I don't want to be sisters with many of those girls. They are just disrespectful of the world and of themselves."

Although my initial impression of belly dancers was that many of the women were surrounded by men in their professional lives, Meredith, like almost half of the dancers I interviewed, works with mostly women. In fact, Meredith and many other dancers in this study are involved in traditionally female-dominated occupations that focus on caring for or supporting others, such as nursing, social work, education, clerical services, and counseling. However, just because women work with other women or are employed in traditionally feminine occupations, does not necessarily translate into strong, positive relationships with female colleagues. Women can hold negative attitudes toward each other in their work settings and exhibit destructive behavior, such as devaluing or sabotaging other women's work, gossiping, excluding women from certain activities, and ignoring female co-workers (Chesler 2001; Tanenbaum 2002). Some belly dancers experience these relatively common issues in the workforce and, as a result, do not seek friendships with their female colleagues. The nature and quality of friendships within one's occupation undoubtedly differs from one's friendships in leisure contexts. In the context of work, people may not build friendships with their co-workers because of some of the negative interactions I described above. Furthermore, it can be difficult for people to form friendships at work because friendships in the workplace can potentially threaten our ability to fully carry out our workplace responsibilities. Therefore, we may not seek to build the same quality of friendships inside the workplace as we do in our leisure activities. Although she is not close to the women at her job, Meredith connects with and enjoys the relationships she builds with women through belly dance.

Like Meredith, Nancy's relationships with her female co-workers are different than the friendships she builds through belly dance. "Part of what I really like about belly dancing is the sisterhood. I work with women, and this is just a different group of women," she continues. "I really like hanging out with the girls in belly dancing because they are my kind of girls," the dancer in her twenties explains. We reaffirm our identity by selective affiliation (Burke and Stets 2009). In other words, we most often chose to spend time with people who confirm our sense of self, whether it is positive or negative. Nancy, like many other belly dancers, associates with other dancers because she views other participants as similar to herself, which together with feeling accepted and supported, results in feelings of "sisterhood."

"Probably friendship" and "the sisterhood of community," Julia replies when I ask her about some of the biggest benefits she gets from belly dance.

"All of my close relationships are with women I dance with," Julia continues. Julia values the sisterhood and community a great deal because "whether or not it's true, so often you hear about or you see on TV and movies, women tearing each other down and not working cooperatively together." Women compete with each other in many areas in life, such as physical appearance, relationships, and work, which can lead to strained relationships between them (Tanenbaum 2002). The women that Julia meets in belly dance "don't act like that and at least make a conscious effort to not act like that and hold each other up and be positive for each other." These women refrain from putting each other down. Instead, they "truly cheer for each other," Julia comments, which is "really important to me." For Julia and many other dancers, belly dance is a refuge from competition and a safe haven to develop close friendships with other women.

Emma found solace with women in belly dance after her divorce. As opposed to other dances, such as ballroom, swing, or salsa, belly dance does not require a partner. Rather, it is a solo dance or a group of individuals. Joining a community in which women do not need men, especially after her marriage dissolved, was very powerful for Emma. "You don't need a man to do it," Emma says. "The empowerment that goes along with it, I think that's the biggest thing," Emma continues. "When you use the word empowerment, what do you mean?" I ask Emma. "Feeling confident," she replies. "You walk in feeling weak and that you need a man to do something. Then you go dance, and it's like, 'you know what I think I'm going to try to change the light bulb,' or you know you just get more self-esteem and confidence," Emma explains.

Emma describes the time she was married: "It was very much him and I. I mean, I had some friends, but it was just like my whole life revolved around him." After she and her husband divorced, Emma recalls that she felt "completely alone." "It was just me and the dogs and cats." Belly dance gave Emma a new social group. Most of the other students in her graduate program are married with children. Many people in Emma's dance class were also graduate students, but most were not married with familial responsibilities. "So that was really cool. I really liked just meeting other single women." "It's very much my peer group," she says.

Like Emma, Scarlett was initially attracted to belly dance because she met a lot of women with whom she had much in common. "There were a lot of similarities I noticed," Scarlett replies when I ask her about the other dancers in her classes. Scarlett felt at ease talking with people she met through belly dance because "I could always find something I had in common with them." Throughout her two years of involvement in belly dance, some of the dancers Scarlett met enjoyed crafting or knitting like she does. Others liked the same kind of music that she did or shared her appreciation of history, especially medieval times.

Although many female belly dancers work with other women, some dancers do not develop close friendships with women at their places of employment. The women that participants meet in belly dance are people with whom they feel connected. Dancers find other people who share similar interests and personality traits. Because they are part of a group with whom they share things in common, belly dance is a site to develop friendships.

"I'm half tomboy and half belly dancer"

Women's friendships are best understood within structural and situational contexts (O'Conner 1992). Many dancers in this study do not have robust social opportunities to build friendships with other women outside of belly dance. In fact, some dancers did not have many girlfriends growing up, so they do not have solid, longstanding childhood relationships to fall back on. Couple these experiences with some of the negative messages women receive from society about the value or quality of female relationships and it is understandable why some belly dancers do not have many strong female friendships outside of the activity. Furthermore, while some belly dancers work primarily with women, a sizable group work primarily with men. Regardless of whether a dancer works with mostly men, some participants have spent most of their time in the company of men. For these women, belly dance is a safe haven from a life that is mostly dominated by men and masculinity.

"Do you have many opportunities to spend time with other women?" I ask Maggie. Other than her female roommate, "I've never been one to hang out with a lot of women," Maggie explains. "But, I've found that a lot of the women I've met in belly dance, I've liked a lot," she continues. "Whereas a lot of the women I've met elsewhere, I've had a harder time bonding with." One reason why Maggie rarely bonds with other women is because "I'm really strange. I'm half tomboy and half belly dancer. I've always been into sports and music, things that girls haven't been into," Maggie tells me. "All of my girlfriends in high school wanted to go shopping all the time, and I was like 'I want to stay home and listen to music.' They were like 'we don't want to do that,'" Maggie recalls. As a result of having different interests from other girls, "I ended up having more guy friends," Maggie explains. Furthermore, Maggie is in a natural sciences graduate program consisting of almost all men. Belly dance gives Maggie an opportunity to participate in more traditionally feminine activities. As Maggie illustrates, women involved in male-dominated graduate programs and work fields seek supportive female relationships outside of school (Aleman 2010).

Shawna also did not spend much time with girls when she was growing up. Belly dance "introduced me to women who were strong and proud on their own and don't feel the need to rip each other to shreds," Shawna tells me. Shawna found women in belly dance who "lift each other to a higher level." Finding women who supported, rather than degraded, each other was really important to Shawna. Since being involved in belly dance for several years, Shawna says, "I finally found women who were strong enough in themselves that they didn't need to hurt someone else." Shawna doesn't have many other outlets to develop friendships with other women because, "I am shy around girls." Now almost thirty, Shawna was twenty-two years old when she developed her first female friendship. "I told my first friend that was a girl that 'I've never had a friend that was a girl before, so you have to help me and tell me when I do something wrong,'" Shawna explains. Shawna did not have female friendships before she was in her twenties partly because she spent a lot of time by herself and, "I get along with guys better than I get along with girls." However, through belly dance, Shawna is "learning how to play well with other girls."

Agnes found a supportive community in belly dance after she was sexually assaulted by a male superior. She came to belly dance about six months after the incident because "it was something physical to do." She was rapidly gaining weight, and she saw belly dance as "this community of women where I thought maybe I could be a little safer than [in] the community of men I just left." Agnes was involved in a physical activity that was dominated by men and stereotypical notions of masculinity, such as physical prowess. She describes this community of mostly men as "aggressive and who want to hit each other in the face." In contrast, at the time she took up belly dance, she viewed the dance as, "let's concentrate on this round fluffy bouncy thing." Joining a new community that she saw as vastly different from the group she left was initially difficult for Agnes. "I had completely not been in touch with that part of myself, that feminine thing," she explains. "Makeup was a complete mystery. I didn't know what I was doing," Agnes confesses. Dancers like Agnes, Maggie, and Shawna spend much of their time surrounded by men. Coming to belly dance offers them an opportunity to form social bonds with other women.

"It's wonderful belonging to something bigger than you"

One goal in ballroom dance is to reach various levels of finals to which some dancers advance, while others do not. Earning a place in a semi or finals competition is so thrilling because not everyone can qualify (Marion 2008). Belly dancers work toward troupe memberships or performance slots in coveted gigs. These opportunities would not be nearly as valuable if they were available to everyone all of the time. For instance, in the summer of 2015, my belly dance troupe performed a five-minute set at Tribal Revolution, arguably the largest tribal belly dance event in the Midwest. Because there is an audition process and this is a high status regional event that only occurs once a year, people in my troupe were ecstatic when we learned we had been selected to perform in one of the evening shows. Preparing for and performing in this show was an intense group effort resulting in a meaningful shared experience.

In her work on relationships between women, Coates's study (1996) shows that collaboration is a powerful way that women do friendship. Belly dancers collaborate in myriad ways. As I described above, they work together to create performances. In addition, they host haflas, and sponsor workshops. A great deal of time and preparation is required for organizing a show. The group may need to find a location for the performance, such as a dance hall. Days, times, and rental prices need to be negotiated. Furthermore, the group may need technicians to help with lighting equipment and speakers. Photographers to take pictures of the event are occasionally hired. If the performance includes live musicians, arrangements for their participation must be made. Advertisements, such as posters, flyers, and Internet postings, need to be disseminated. Decisions regarding who will be responsible for ticket sales and admission need to be made.

Rehearsing for shows also takes a lot of time. Some acts require dancers to develop or learn choreography and different dancers are assigned individual parts that contribute to the performance. If the dance is an American Tribal Style performance, participants depend on a lead dancer to give them cues about which movements to execute. The lead dancer who is being followed must clearly execute her movements so the followers are able to mimic the movements. In these cases, dancers depend on each other to follow movements and dance cues, which require much practice and time dancing together. "It's one thing to make friends but another thing to be a part of something bigger," Emma proclaims. As part of a group of dancers who take classes and perform together at various community events, Emma continues, "the troupe is the bigger thing and doing things to contribute to that group [is important to her]" rather than just having a few friends to hang out with.

Larissa considers belly dance to be more communal than other physical activities, such as aerobics classes. In aerobics classes, and some other forms of exercise, participants rarely share a common goal beyond losing weight or building muscle tone. Even in these cases, the goals are ultimately achieved by individual participants. For example, Larissa had fun in a body sculpting class she took, but she felt isolated. "It is kind of you working out by yourself, and you working on you," Larissa explains. However, during her belly dance lessons, especially the performance class she takes, "you are all helping each other learn . . . you are working for a common goal."

One of the primary reasons why belly dance is a place for women to develop friendships with one another is because it is relatively cooperative and non-hierarchical, which contrasts with the competitive nature of many work environments. In work situations, there are various levels of management and bosses setting goals for their employees. In order to effectively manage their staff, managers may be leery of developing close friendships with their workers. Likewise, workers may be set up in a competition with each other for promotions, raises, and other accolades. Contrasting work settings, the structure of many leisure activities, such as belly dance, is less competitive and more equal. The somewhat flat structure of belly dance provides a place for participants to work together toward common goals, which can help support feelings of community and the formation of friendships. One of the reasons why belly dance is so special for Trisha is that it "is not a competitive group of women." Rather, it is a "very consensus driven group of women," Trisha explains. Trisha contrasts the consensus building that she sees in belly dance with her job. She works with mostly men in an information technology position. "Women like to get a consensus," Trisha suggests. However, "guys are much more hierarchical." She continues, "I spend all day working with guys in a business environment that is a very classic business structure." Trisha describes her place of business as a "very conservative company" with directors, managers, and "chains of command." Trisha's place of employment operates very much like a "pyramid shaped business structure." In lieu of the top-down model of decision-making that Trisha experiences at her job, in her belly dance group, "they are all going to talk about it and arrive at something that works for everybody." Trisha sadly adds, "Eighty hours a week of mine are not spent in that environment at all."

None of the male dancers with whom I spoke talked about "brotherhood" as a primary benefit of being involved in the dance. Scholarship on male and female friendships shows that women's friendships with other women are more intimate than men's friendships (Freysinger 1995). Women's participation in leisure centers on their relationships with others to a greater degree than men's participation in leisure (Freysinger 1995). In contrast, studies show that in same-sex friendships, men focus on the activity and doing things with their male friends more than forming interpersonal connections (Aukett *et al.* 1988; Williams, 1985). Due to the dearth of male participants in American belly dance, this activity is not a site to examine same-sex male friendships. However, I find that male belly dancers value community and feelings of belonging in ways that are not illuminated in earlier work on same-sex male friendships.

As an ATS dancer, Phil appreciates the group nature of his dance. "One moment you're in control, and the next moment someone else is in control," Phil comments as he describes the follow-the-leader format of ATS dancing. "You are creating that beauty, but you aren't creating it alone," Phil remarks. Not only does Phil appreciate the collective nature of ATS dance, but he acknowledges that every member of the group must work together to create an effective and attractive ATS performance.

"I would definitely say the sense of a tribe, a community of people that are all interested in this ethnic art form," Mark replies when I ask him about the benefits he gets from the dance. What helps dancers feel like they are part of a community is the distinct language spoken within their dance circles. In this sense, belly dance is similar to a club or organization about which not everyone has insider knowledge.

"I know the language"

"You mentioned that the improvisation of tribal was important to you. What is it about improvisation that you like?" I ask Agnes. "It's a communication between the dancers," Agnes replies without hesitation. Agnes contrasts her tribal improvisational dancing with some choreographed cabaret group dances. When she participates in a planned cabaret dance, "it is always like one, two, three, step ball change, five, six, seven, eight. Crap! I'm in the wrong spot," Agnes laughs. Agnes continues, "You really are inside your own head, and I never got to the point in cabaret when I could tune in with the audience, the music, and with my fellow dancers." However, when Agnes dances the tribal style, "you have certain moves and everybody that speaks the tribal language knows these moves, so when you get together with people and you have a common language, you can have a conversation." Agnes believes this conversation "takes place on a stage and with music that is so different than sitting down over coffee." "It's an amazingly powerful thing," Agnes says. "There are leaders and followers, but everyone takes a turn leading. It's an incredibly joyful performance," Agnes concludes. As Agnes demonstrates, the structure of some tribal dance may be particularly conducive to developing friendships through the communal rules and interconnections required to successfully execute the movements.

Although Alicia does not frequently participate in belly dance, she connects with other dancers. "How do you feel connected to other dancers?" I wonder. Echoing Agnes, she replies, "They all speak the same language." This common vocabulary became evident to Alicia when she attended a regional belly dance gathering and there were "all these women from different states, different cities, and with different dance [backgrounds]," Alicia explains. Although the focus of the event is on tribal dance, Alicia recognizes that "Tribal can mean so many things." She describes a workshop she attended at which participants were paired together. "I had a really awesome partner who was an Egyptian dancer. Dance wise we didn't have a lot in common, but we had belly dance as a base. That was what we were there for. It was an instant connection," Alicia explains. So unlike Agnes who feels connected to other tribal dancers with whom she shares a language, Alicia's bond with another dancer was not limited to a particular style of belly dance. Rather, they connected over their shared appreciation of belly dance.

Sally has an on-and-off relationship with belly dance. She started taking lessons about a year and a half ago, stopped, started again, and stopped. Even though she was not taking dance classes or performing when we talk, she feels connected to the belly dance community. Similar to Alicia's sentiments, Sally connects with other dancers based on a shared language, including names of dance moves and musical patterns. "Some of my friendships with belly dancers have been better because I know the language," Sally explains. "I can understand what they are talking about even though I am not doing it . . . When I say taqsim [pronounced tock-seem], you know what I am talking about." But the people Sally works with do not know that language. "When I talk about it at work, they all think I'm a nut. 'So taqsim, is that like a taxi?'" Sally jokes. Although she does not actively participate in belly dance anymore, Sally maintains her friendships with people in the belly dance community and "because I can share [the language] with them and have actually done it, I've gotten closer to my friends." Because every group has its own idioculture, group members distinguish themselves from outsiders partly by their shared language (Fine 1979). Knowing a language that is only shared within a certain community bonds people together and gives them a feeling of status, at least within that particular community.

Two worldwide belly dance flash mob events illustrate the value of shared language and community. Every year since 2007, on the designated World Belly Dance Day (second Saturday in May), dancers all over the globe dance the same choreography to the same music wearing the same T-shirt. In 2014, dancers in more than 200 cities on five continents participated in this event (see shimmymob.com). In 2012, members of the ATS community created a similar yearly event that occurs on the second Saturday in October. Since ATS is not a choreographed form of dance, the ATS Flash Mob designates a common song, but not a set of movements (see ATS Flash Mob Facebook page). Both the Shimmy Mob and ATS Flash Mob occur in any location the participants wish, such as a mall, street, event, or home. Many participants in both mobs record their dance and post it on various Internet sites. In the case of the Shimmy Mob, dancers connect with others all over the world by dancing the same choreography. With the ATS Flash Mob, dancers marvel at their shared knowledge of movements performed by others across the globe. "I had no idea how it would turn out and when I started seeing the responses and then all the videos come rolling in from all over the world, I was moved to tears. I still am every year," Heidi Capps-Hayden, the creator of the ATS Flash Mob, tells me. "What is it that moves you to tears?" I ask. "One world united in dance.

The spirit and heart of it. The beauty. The joy . . . It just radiates an energy that touches me." In other words, to paraphrase Heidi, the event unites people from around the world into one global community.

Reflections on friendships in belly dance

As the song ends, the seven of us form a straight line facing the audience, join hands, raise our arms, and bow in unison signaling the end of our unusually long twelve-minute dance performance. One after another, we gracefully walk away from the performance area with our hands gently resting on our hips. The moment that Terri is out of the audience's site, she cradles her face in her hands and begins to cry. She is moving out of the state in a few weeks and this is her final performance with our troupe. "I knew I was going to cry the second I left the stage," Terri quietly tells us. Several of the dancers begin to wipe away their own tears. We all take turns giving our dance sister a tight hug. We know we will miss her as much as she will miss us, and we don't know when we will see her again. After we have each given her a hug, we form a circle for one large group embrace.

"You ladies mean the world to me," Terri later tells me. Out of the many family and friends that Terri informed she was moving, the members of our dance group "were the hardest of my local friends to tell," she continues. It is deeply moving to Terri that "we were [our instructor's] first students here and we formed the student troupe together. It's going to be so hard leaving you," Terri tells me. Creating the troupe and the work we did together learning and performing provided many structural opportunities for Terri to build deep friendships within our dance community. These bonds became some of the most important relationships that Terri formed in the area, rendering it especially emotional for her and her troupe when she moved.

Friendships are not something that we have. They are something that we do. There are several mechanisms within belly dance that support the development of close friendships. The costumes and performance aspect of belly dance help some dancers overcome their shyness and introverted tendencies, which contributes to them being more social and supports their developing friendships. Also, norms dictate that dancers support, encourage, and accept each other, and those values are sometimes enforced when lines are crossed. Furthermore, because belly dance is a social world with a common culture that is not available to many people outside of the pursuit, dancers feel connected to each other through a shared knowledge and language. Finally, belly dance is a relatively non-hierarchical leisure space, which supports cooperation among dancers. In this space, participants meet others who are like-minded and share their interests.

Although a sense of community matters to them, not one of the men with whom I spoke emphasized friendship as a primary benefit of participating in belly dance. The development and maintenance of friendships appears to be more relevant and central for women's experiences within the dance compared to the men. In fact, the friendships that women make within the belly dance community are so important that when some dancers leave the community, they sometimes profoundly miss those relationships. After being involved in belly dance for less than five years, Lilly ceased her participation in the dance. She moved to another state, started a new job, and was in the process of getting acclimated to a new area. "I miss the community and friendships," Lilly tells me. When she was actively involved in belly dance, she danced at local clubs with some of her dance friends as one might expect of someone in her twenties and in college. Since she has graduated and moved out of the state, Lilly does not have the opportunity to go dancing with her friends. "I definitely think belly dancing has made me miss my female friendships, which are important," Lilly continues. Like so many of the other dancers discussed in this chapter, Lilly had closer male friends in high school and college. At that time in her life she thought women "didn't want to be friends with me for some reason." So the friends she made through belly dance were that much more meaningful to her. "The ladies from the troupe were the first time I had so many female friends, and that was great. I made that bond."

Chapter 5

A spiritual dance

It's a Saturday evening. A few street lights stream in through the windows of the auditorium on the first floor of the recreation center. The room is dark with no overhead lighting. Folding metal chairs are arranged on each side of the elongated tile floor to create a middle aisle. Slow, melodic music plays over the speakers. Through a door in the back of the open space, the eight of us gradually step single file down the center of the room as we slowly make our way toward the stage. Our long black skirts and pants are nearly camouflaged by the darkness of the room, while our tops and belts covered with silver fringe and metal sparkle against flickering candle light. In each of our hands, we hold rounded, slightly opaque deep orange jars that cradle a small candle. We gingerly step forward to preserve the flame. A subtle stream of smoke rises from our jars as a musty scent surrounds us. As we reach the stage, we divide into two groups. From both sides of the stage, we climb the five steps, careful not to step on our skirts. When we all reach the stage, we form a semi-circle on the elevated platform facing the sea of chairs and the audience.

As the soft, melodic music continues, we gently raise and lower our arms while twisting our wrists to move the candle jars up and down and around our bodies. I feel nervous about accidentally extinguishing my candle or, even worse, setting something on fire. I anxiously clutch my jar to ensure that I will not drop the candle or prematurely blow out the light. I have a tendency to be a klutz, so I intensely focus on protecting myself, my costume, and my fellow dancers from the candle flame. At the same time, I feel incredibly relaxed and calm as I join my dance sisters in the relatively simple movements. For a few minutes, I forget there is an audience gazing upon us. I am mesmerized by the candlelight, and the rhythmic music without lyrics soothes me. Stepping my feet, swaying my hips from right to left, and my awareness of the bright candles juxtaposed against the dark auditorium becomes a moving meditation for me. As the song begins to fade, we step forward and form a line near the front of the stage. Together we bring our knees to the floor, and in unison, blow out our candles, leaving a darkened room.

I danced this routine during one of my very first belly dance performances. It was and remains one of the few dances that brought me into a state that I might call spiritual. The combination of low lighting, soft glowing candles, and slow and simple music lacking any distinguishable words becomes very meditative for me. Every time I practice or perform this dance, I slip into a trance-like state. The experience is hypnotic. My involvement in this dance partly contributed to my curiosity about a broader connection between belly dance and spirituality.

This chapter explores why and how many participants construct spiritual meaning within belly dance. I address spirituality because people increasingly are creating spiritual meaning in their everyday lives, which is sometimes referred to as "lived" religion (McGuire 2008). Lived religious practices may draw from mainstream religious communities (Ammerman 1987), and they may also occur in mundane settings outside of traditional religious boundaries (Ammerman 2007; Bender 2010; McGuire 1988). Some people associate spirituality with a wide variety of leisure activities, such as being in nature, reading, walking and running, traveling, and playing a variety of sports (Schmidt and Little 2007; Williams 2010). Along with such leisure pursuits, some people also create spiritual experiences through a myriad of artistic outlets, such as music, painting, sculpting (Wuthnow 2001), and singing (McGuire 2008). Belly dance is one artistic leisure site that offers a variety of tools that many participants use to infuse the activity with spiritual meaning in highly creative ways. Furthermore, considering spirituality sheds light on gender dynamics within belly dance because there is a large mythos surrounding female-centered spiritual roots and belly dance. Along with considering whether and how this mythos has any relevance for female dancers today, it is also meaningful to consider how men navigate spirituality within an activity that is heavily dominated by women.

Embodied spirituality and dance

Some artistic expressions of spirituality involve the body (McGuire 2003a, 2003b). Bodies help us experience the world around us through our senses, such as touch, sound, and sight. Bodily movements, such as posture and gestures, are used to create spiritual experiences (McGuire 2003b, 2007). Physical movements can enhance spiritual practices by helping the practitioner access inner emotions and deep insights about one's life (Sointu and Woodhead 2008).

Dance is one type of artistic embodied practice during which some people use their bodies for spiritual expression (Zinnbauer et al. 1999; Stewart 2000; Shira 2000). It has been argued that dance reunites body, soul, and mind and heightens consciousness (Stewart 2000). As a spiritual practice, dance can serve as prayer or worship (Wuthnow 2001, 2003) and produce individual "highs" that transcend everyday occurrences (Flinn 1995). In fact, Wiccans use several bodily practices, including dance, to enter a religious trance (Salomensen

2002). Dance may also aid a participant in establishing a deep connection, either within him/herself or with a higher power (Wuthnow 2001, 2003). People may also use dance to uncover and express deep emotions, communicate joy, and produce a sense of community and connectedness (Foltz 2006; McGuire 2007; Takahashi and Olaveson 2003). People infuse a variety of dance forms with spiritual meaning, including ballet (Aalten 2004), African dance (Monteiro and Wall 2011), Afro-Cuban Santeria (Hagedorn 2001), samba (Browning 1995), classical Asian dance (Shay 2008), electronic dance or raves (Beck and Lynch 2009; Hutson 2000; Takahashi and Olaveson 2003), and country dance (Flinn 1995). Belly dance is another form of dance that is spiritually meaningful for many of its participants (Crosby 2000; Dox 2005; Jorgensen 2012; Kraus 2009; Moe 2012; Sellers-Young 1992).

Because belly dance is a commonplace activity not formally connected to a religious organization, I use the term "spirituality," rather than religion, to discuss the experiences of some dancers. Furthermore, I do not rely on a single, predetermined definition of spirituality. People have different understandings of spirituality (Ammerman 2007, 2010), and I do not want to disregard a dancer's experience that she or he may define as spiritual just because that occurrence may not fit with a particular definition of spirituality. I ask dancers whether and how they experience spirituality within belly dance however they define this concept for themselves. As we shall see, although belly dance is spirituality meaningful for many dancers, what that spirituality means, how it is constructed, and the circumstances under which people create it varies greatly.

Emergent spirituality

Experiencing spirituality in belly dance is one of the foundational reasons why some participants enter this dance world. They were either searching for a spiritual home or the spirituality they found in belly dance was so profoundly meaningful to them that they wanted to become more involved in the activity. The first time Phil experienced spirituality was a major factor in pushing him to get more involved in belly dance. He likens his spirituality in belly dance to tarab in Arab culture, which Phil describes as "spirits channeling through you when you dance." The first time Phil experienced tarab "is why I started dancing." It occurred during a warm summer evening when he stood around a fire watching people dance. The moon shone bright as drummers pounded out various rhythms. After observing people dance for about an hour, someone approached Phil and encouraged him to join the dancers. Phil remembers:

> After five minutes, the fire melted away. It wasn't there anymore. The other people weren't there anymore. All I could hear was the drums. This energy was

there and when I came out of it, it was three hours later. It's kind of frightening because I'm usually in control of my life most of the time, and I wasn't in control at that moment. I have no clue what happened.

Unlike dancers who set spiritual intentions within Afro-Cuban Santeria (Hagedorn 2001), "my spirituality is something that is given to me. I have no control over my spirituality," Phil explains. "I think I've danced all these years because I long for the moment to have that opportunity again, and it really is a gift. You don't get it all the time," Phil continues. Phil has only experienced tarab four times over his twenty years of involvement in this dance. His first occurrence with spirituality was so profound that Phil wanted to become more involved in belly dance and has stayed with it for over two decades partly hoping for additional spiritual experiences. What is it about belly dance that some people construct it as spiritually meaningful?

Getting "lost" in the music

We use music to sustain and enhance how we view ourselves. Music can block internal or external noise and drown out distractions so people can immerse themselves in the present. Different pieces of music resonate with varying aspects of our lives and experiences. In this way, music can help people shift moods and achieve desired physical, psychological, and mental states. For instance, slow music can help people relax and feel a sense of peace (DeNora 2000).

Music is one of the primary components of belly dance that participants use to facilitate spiritual expression. Some belly dance incorporates Middle Eastern tunes, and the lyrics are not always understandable to American dancers. When people do not focus on the words, they may be better able to lose themselves in the music, which is conducive for having a spiritual experience. For example, reciting a Latin prayer at a Roman Catholic mass or chanting Hebrew in a Jewish synagogue may facilitate a spiritual experience for native English speakers. Many dancers attach spiritual meaning to belly dance when they get "lost" or "zone out," which is typically facilitated by the music.

Listening to certain songs helps Alicia let go of her everyday concerns. She especially likes dancing to Middle Eastern fusion music. Although she doesn't mind dancing to other types of music, "it doesn't bring that same type of [spiritual] feeling as when I am dancing to Middle Eastern music," Alicia explains. Because she doesn't understand Middle Eastern song lyrics, "I don't focus on the words." But when she dances to music with words that she knows, her experience changes, and she gets distracted by the words. Alicia comments further, "I really like to dance to music that has no singing in it . . . I just hear the melody and the rhythm . . . I tune in more with the emotion rather than the words if I don't understand them."

Escaping into music is similar to entering a meditative zone or trance during which participants become completely absorbed in the activity and forget about everything else going on around them. "There is sort of a zone you could get into when dancing to a good piece of music. I think that verges on being a spiritual experience if you are broadly defining it. It is meditative where you get that kind of Zen-like trance," Trisha explains. The music that accompanies their belly dance allows some dancers like Trisha to create spiritual experiences within the dance. Some dance scholars refer to this experience as flow (Jorgensen 2012).

"In flow, people experience a sense of complete mastery over their environment as well as an intense and focused attention on the activity" (Carpentier et al. 2012:504). Outside distractions and concerns melt away and the activity is the only thing on which a person in flow focuses. Typically, flow is achieved when there is balance between challenge in an activity and mastery over it. Therefore, people who achieve flow typically have some level of competency in their given activity (Csikszentmihalyi and Hunter 2003). Peg has been involved in belly dance for over seven years, so she has some level of dance competency. She equates spirituality in belly dance with ritual in Catholicism. "You go in and you know exactly what's going to happen. If you want to, you can lose yourself in the movement and connect with the divine because you know exactly what is going to happen and you can feel the flow of the ritual." In other words, dancers like Peg can get lost in the dance and music when they are familiar enough with movements and the song that they do not have to concentrate on what they need to do next.

Dancing, as a form of ritual, can move people out of ordinary consciousness and into an altered state (Magliocco 2004). Salomonsen (2002:209) defines ritualization as "the intentional interaction between social bodies and ritually defined structured space in order to induce change or confirmation in the ritualists." Basic principles of ritual include the body acting in some space. Ritual can be fluid and improvisational within some kind of structure, such as the structure of particular movements (Magliocco 2004). Scarlett, for example, experiences spirituality in belly dance when her experiences are ritualistic and formally set up. "It's all because you are in the clothes and right place and mood and the setting contributes to that. There's something about doing it with people that sort of adds to it," Scarlett tells me. For dancers like Scarlett, a structured belly dance environment with props, music, and other people is conducive to creating spiritual experiences because they help focus one's attention on the dance and unrelated distractions are minimized. Similarly, the "Spiral Dance" is a common Wiccan ritual performed around Halloween. Much like Scarlett's analogy to ritual, the Spiral Dance involves the creation of sacred space via the presence of drummers, dim lights, incense, and the sprinkling of water (Salomonsen 2002). Both the Wiccan Spiral Dance and belly dance as ritual are constructed using various props in particular settings with specific people that support feelings of spirituality.

"It's kind of like a drug"

Many participants believe that belly dance is spiritual because it is a mental escape. Rather than thinking about home or work or other areas of life that may be causing participants to feel stress, dancers focus on properly executing moves, keeping a beat with the rhythm, and putting moves together into a coherent and smooth dance. For Scarlett, belly dance is a break away from unease and over thinking. As a graduate student in her mid-twenties, Scarlett explains that she usually feels anxious. "I'm always thinking. My brain doesn't stop," Scarlett says. "When I belly dance, I feel more serene, and I'm not thinking about anything. It's the only time when I'm not thinking," Scarlett tells me. She continues:

> My whole anal personality gets shifted to belly dancing. Now instead of focusing on words and semicolons, I'm focusing on joints and angles and foot posturing, but it seems different because it's not mental. My job and everything is so mental, and so much of it happens in my head.

Belly dance movements differ from standard American dancing. To maintain proper posture and correctly execute the movements, dancers must train their bodies to move in new ways. They engage muscles in their torso, chest, back, and shoulders that the general public does not use on a regular basis, which requires a certain level of concentration and communication with their body (Stewart 2000). In this way, the embodied nature of belly dance facilitates spiritual experiences for some dancers.

Like Scarlett, belly dance "keeps me sane," Gwen says. "How does it keep you sane?" I ask. "It helps give me a break from math. [Belly dance helps me use] a completely different side of my brain. Sometimes, if I get stuck on a problem, I'll just dance for a little while and then go back to work on it," Gwen replies. "I think everybody needs an outlet. People jog to clear their mind. People read books. Everybody needs something. For me, it is dance," Gwen explains. In this way, belly dance is not unlike gym-goers who use the gym as a way to take their minds off everyday concerns (Crossley 2006a); they engage in an activity that allows them to take a break from their everyday existence.

Scarlett and Gwen's experiences are similar to the tango "high." Savigliano (1998) describes the tango "high" as the state that people reach where they feel grounded and at ease. They abandon their mental concerns while maintaining full control over their body. In the same way, belly dancers do not abandon their dance structure or form. While maintaining their dance steps, dancers leave their mental cares behind and focus solely on the dance, as Scarlett suggested.

Like the tango high, several belly dancers suggest they get an emotional high or adrenalin rush from belly dance. "It is kind of like a drug," Denny tells me one evening after he finishes his dance class. "Like today . . . It was such a rush! Let's do that again!" Denny says. Likening his feelings to a high that one might receive from a mind-altering substance is similar to what Cohen and Taylor (1992) call "mindscaping." Rather than altering one's physical surroundings, mindscaping is one form of escape from everyday life in which people use drugs to mentally take a break and change what happens in their heads (Cohen and Taylor 1992). Although they are not using mind-altering substances, dancers like Scarlett, Gwen, and Denny believe belly dance is spiritual because their participation allows them to mentally escape from their ordinary routines.

"I am getting more comfortable with myself"

When we step out of the continuity of life, we sometimes participate in leisure pursuits that provide a safe space for identity work and self-expression (Cohen and Taylor 1992). These activities allow us to temporarily escape the repetitiveness of everyday life and renegotiate identity with a fresh set of resources that we may not have available to us in our regular existence. We take these new resources, reconstruct our sense of self, and apply these tools to refresh identities in our everyday lives (Cohen and Taylor 1992). This experience is like George Simmel's (1971) concept of the "adventurer" who temporarily drops out of everyday routines. Our experiences in an adventure give new meanings to our everyday worlds and provide a new perspective so that we may return to our lives rejuvenated (Simmel 1971).

People can use a new set of tools available within their activity enclaves to renegotiate their sense of self, which can result in a personal transformation (Cohen and Taylor 1992; Simmel 1971). A spirituality associated with personal transformation occurs when people attempt to heal some emotional and/or physical aspect of themselves (Cimino and Lattin 2002; Moberg 2000; Roof 1999; Woods and Ironson 1999). This healing involves creating a sense of wholeness or reaching into a dimension of one's higher self (Woods and Ironson 1999; Fuller 2001). Belly dance helps some people express and feel good about themselves, develop a deeper self-understanding, and feel more content with their lives.

As a self-proclaimed shy person, Abigail uses belly dance to help her feel more socially secure. "I guess [belly dance] just really makes me feel connected with my body, how I think about myself, and how I think about how I fit into the world around me, which is spirituality," Abigail tells me. Abigail continues, "Coming into belly dancing, I wasn't really comfortable with my own skin, and I wasn't very good at connecting with other people . . . I am getting more comfortable with myself, accepting of how I am and who I am."

Abigail's focus on feeling more connected to her body is not unlike George Herbert Mead's (1934) concept of fusing the "I" and "me." According to Mead, the "I" and "me" are two intertwining moments of an act. Briefly, the "me" refers to our ability to adopt the attitudes of other people, understand the interrelationships between people, and possess knowledge of our communities. Mead refers to this social knowledge as the generalized other. The "me" allows us to take the role of this other and see ourselves and the world from the position of the other. The "I" refers to how we act based on our understanding of other people, relationships, and knowledge. Mead argues there are some situations in which the "I" and "me" are fused together and result in "exaltation" or an "intense emotional experience" (Mead 1934: 273–274).

According to Mead (1934), intense emotional responses are frequently located in religious activities. When we experience this "exaltation" within religion, we feel a strong sense of belonging and community, much like what Durkheim (1912) identifies. We completely and thoroughly identify with other members of our community and, like the three musketeers, we experience a sense of "all for one and one for all." In other words, our interests and the interests of those in our community merge. These "precious" experiences, as Mead refers to them, allow us to feel "at one" with everyone around us and at peace with everything about ourselves. In belly dance, spiritual experiences partly include the connection between the mind and body that contributes to these types of "precious" experiences described by Mead. For some participants, such as Abigail, belly dance facilitates a merger of the mind and body, resulting in some dancers feeling more whole, which can lead to feelings of exaltation and spirituality. Furthermore, feeling more comfortable with themselves helps facilitate connection with other people.

"I feel a real connectedness with the people I am dancing with"

Spirituality consists of connections between an individual and a community of like-spirited individuals (Ammerman 2010, 2013; Foltz 2006; McGuire 2003b, 2007; Zinnbauer *et al.* 1999; Zinnbauer and Pargament 2005). According to Émile Durkheim (1912), a religion comes into being and is legitimated through what he calls "collective effervescence." Collective effervescence refers to moments in social life when a group of individuals comes together, communicates similar thoughts, and participates in the same action, which serves to unify the group. During these times, a certain electricity is created and released, leading participants to a high degree of collective emotional excitement or delirium. This impersonal, extra-individual force, which is a core element of religion, transports the individuals into a new, ideal realm, lifts them up outside of themselves, and makes them feel as if they are in contact with an extraordinary energy (Durkheim 1912).

Being part of a community, such as group classes, or extended communities where people are involved in the same activity but are not physically together, can produce a spiritual connection (Stanczak 2006). Some participants use belly dance to create those kinds of spiritual connections with other people from previous generations or in the present, such as audience members, other dancers, musicians, and general humanity. The spirituality that Lydia associates with belly dance is not "bigger" than her. Lydia creates a horizontal, rather than vertical, spiritual connection that spans history. For Lydia, belly dance "has a timeless quality . . . It's connecting with something that's feminine and very old and a way of feeling that I think all women can relate to." Lydia's experiences are similar to people who participate in a variety of "exotic" dance forms, such as Latin America and classical Asian dances (Shay 2008). By participating in these dance styles, people feel connected to members of ethnic groups that differ from their own who have been involved in these dances throughout history.

Along with connecting to women from previous generations, belly dance also helps some dancers establish connections with other people who attend a belly dance event, such as people in the audience, live musicians, and other dancers. As a partner dance, the tango "high" is occasionally achieved when there is a complete symmetry and connection between the two dancers (Savigliano 1998). Abigail first experienced spirituality in belly dance when she started choreographing and performing duets with a good friend of hers who was also in her dance troupe. Abigail tells me about a particular dance they performed one evening after a workshop. "It went really well. We hit all our cues, and I think we have a good energy between us," she says. Many of their friends in the troupe enjoy watching Abigail and her friend dance together because "we have a good connection and energy between us. I think that really came through to the audience that night," Abigail explains.

Emma believes that dancing American Tribal Style facilitates spiritual connections more than other dance styles. "It's all about healing and doing a ritual," Emma comments about her dance group. "I don't really get [spiritual] with cabaret, just [her specific group] and tribal." Her group and tribal dancing in general are "more about connection with people and Amcab [American cabaret] is more individual . . . With tribal you feel more of a connection to community . . . With Amcab it is just about yourself . . . To me that [connection] is more spiritual." Emma's group formed after the September 11, 2001 attacks. "They did the walk through New York to promote healing and sending positive energy," Emma continues. When Emma dances with her group "it would be that mindset of promoting strength and sending out good messages to the world . . . doing something for social causes versus just being goofy," she comments. Although Emma's group focuses on helping other people, she considers other forms of belly dance to be somewhat superficial and focused on having fun rather than wanting to make a difference in other people's lives.

Like Emma, Phil is also an American Tribal Style dancer. Although he loves dancing in a group, and it is the primary reason why he enjoys ATS, he has not experienced spirituality when dancing this style. On one hand, ATS dancing may be more conducive to creating connections between dancers (as Emma suggests) partly because of the interdependence between dancers. On the other hand, this style requires a level of concentration that may be more prohibitive to dancers entering a spiritual state. Because dancers are connected to and dependent on one another, followers cannot slip into their own world because they will no longer be focused on the leader and will lose track of which movements to execute. Likewise, leaders need to concentrate on clearly performing movements and giving clear cues so the other dancers can follow them. "I never got tarab out of ATS. Only as a soloist. I've had good dances, but never tarab," Phil tells me. Phil has only experienced spirituality when he dances solo. Furthermore, the presence of live musicians is crucial for the few times he has experienced spirituality while dancing. Although there may be hundreds of people watching him, "I've faded away into this moment that's not grounded," Phil explains about his spiritual experiences. Despite all of the people in the audience, "all there is the drummer, the music, and the movement." Although audiences are present during the times Phil remembers experiencing spirituality, he loses awareness of them.

Along with developing spiritual connections with their fellow dancers and musicians, a few dancers also feel spiritually with their students and audience members during performances. Agnes comments, "On stage, you're creating something. You're reaching outside of yourself, and you're handing your heart to your troupe mates and to the audience." This spiritual back and forth that Agnes experiences with audiences also sometimes occurs when she is in a dance classroom. Agnes elaborates:

When you're teaching, things change because as much as you're telling someone what you know, they're telling you what they know. So there is an exchange going on. If you're handing them your heart and spirit, they're handing you theirs. That's amazing that you can get that kind of communication with another human being . . . You're grounding, you're centering, you're shining and you're receiving a gift that is amazing. I don't see how that can't be spiritual.

Many dancers experience meaningful connections with a variety of other people through belly dance, such as fellow dancers, musicians, and audience members. The feelings they get from these experiences are so strong that many dancers infuse these experiences with spiritual significance.

Belly dance is a path to "commune with the mother goddess and father god"

Along with various interpersonal connections that dancers feel with other people in a belly dance scene, many participants also feel a stronger bond with an entity larger than themselves, such as a universal energy or higher power. Some female dancers invoke a feminine goddess that serves as a guide for their personas while dancing (Crosby 2000; Dox 2005; Stewart 2000). About the goddess archetypes she invokes in her dance, Peg says, "My favorite is Bast or Bastet, the Egyptian cat goddess . . . She's one of my matrons." "When I do an archetype performance, I bring her essence into me and part of my perfor-mance is very cat like, very predator like, very slinky on the stage. She is this mother goddess. She's very comforting," Peg explains. "So this is the spiritual connection with how I dance . . . If I want to honor the divine, I dance," Peg continues. Like Peg and some other belly dancers, some samba dancers call on a goddess's power (Browning 1995) and Wiccans occasionally invoke the god-dess by using some anthropomorphic image or symbol (Salomonsen 2002).

Similar to other Wiccans (Salomensen 2002), Nick incorporates both god-dess and god symbols into his spiritual practice. "One way to commune with the mother goddess and father god is through physical act. When you dance, and I think this is true for a lot of dancers, it's like you go to a more primal level of yourself . . . To me, when you get dancing on the spiritual side, you start communing," Nick explains. "I think one reason why I started enjoying it so much was because, and this goes back to the spirituality, I hated my job. I was in a bad place, and I wasn't being very spiritual. I started dancing," Nick continues. "I got back to dancing and felt that there were other things to think about or to be concerned with other than OK when I get into work, I have to get a report done by ten o'clock because it has to get to the director or what-ever," Nick elaborates. Similar to men who use leisure pursuits as escapes from their ordinary lives (Hunt 2008; Schwalbe 1996) and people who run partly because they are dissatisfied with their jobs (Altheide and Pfuhl 1980), belly dance provides a spiritual and welcomed break from Nick's job that he "hated."

Obstacles to spirituality

Similar to the variety of experiences and beliefs that foster spirituality, various cognitive barriers block participants from infusing belly dance with spiritual meaning. Some dancers construct meanings of belly dance that are incompatible with their understandings of spirituality. Many of these definitions involve outside distractions that render spiritual meaning-making difficult.

Alternative definitions of belly dance

When dancers define the act of belly dance as an entertaining performance or as a social/folk dance (as opposed to art), they are not as likely to infuse their experiences with spiritual meaning. Dena is better able to create spiritual experiences when dancing in her home compared to when she is focused on entertaining an audience. "I think [belly dance is] not spiritual when you are performing because you need to think of the audience. Are you connecting with them?" Dena wonders aloud. Earlier, I discussed how many dancers experience spirituality in belly dance when they lose themselves in the activity. But when Dena performs, "You can't just listen to the music and let it go. You need to already have done that work at home, and once you have a performance, you have an audience to worry about." Being attuned to her audience means scanning the crowd and identifying who may be most interested in her dancing for them. Dancing alone allows Dena to express herself freely and enter a particular mental space without the pressures of entertaining an audience. As Dena illustrates, some dancers consider spirituality to be intrinsic, and when they share the dance with others, the activity becomes extrinsic.

In the rare occurrences in which performing is spiritually meaningful for Dena, she feels surrounded by a supportive and appreciative audience whom she does not feel pressure to entertain. Dena comments:

> When I have had a spiritual experience, [it was when] my friend and I used to dance at a little place . . . four shows a night. There was never anyone at the last show. Sometimes we'd dance just for the people who worked there or just for ourselves. That can become almost spiritual. It can be spiritual because you are dancing for people who you know appreciate what you are doing and you don't have to entertain them. You are just dancing and they are just watching . . . For one thing, you get a lot of approval-feedback as opposed to when you are dancing for the standard general public . . . [Feedback from the general public] tends to be entertainment feedback rather than appreciating what they have seen feedback.

94

Dena, and many other dancers, do not infuse belly dance with spiritual meaning when they define themselves as entertainers. "It's a dance. A folk dance," Henry says. "I'm sometimes offended by people who say belly dance is a goddess dance. My dance is not a goddess dance," he explains. "What is offensive?" I ask. "They are saying that the dance I'm doing is part of their ritual. No, the dance I'm doing is entertainment. It's not ritual. There are particular rituals that can be done, but that's not what belly dance is," Henry continues. "It's not a mother ritual. It's not a goddess ritual." Henry draws clear boundaries around dance as entertainment and spirituality. Rather than a mother or goddess ritual, Henry refers to belly dance as a "movement vocabulary" that he traces back to Jamila and Suhaila Salimpour whom he claims learned dance by watching movies, not by watching rituals.

Like Henry, Andy defines belly dance as primarily a folk or social dance, so his definition is also incompatible with his understanding of spirituality. Andy believes that attaching spiritual meaning to belly dance is something reserved primarily for female American Tribal Style dancers. "Is belly dance spiritual for you?" I ask the dancer who is in his sixties. "Not a bit," Andy quickly retorts. "I think it's another thing they do with the ATS. They talk about this spirituality of women united and blah blah blah," Andy continues. "No, that's not for me. It's still like the folk dance in Egypt. Everyone, the men, women, the children, the dogs would start dancing around . . . It's a family thing to express joy," Andy says. Rather than spirituality, when I ask Andy what benefits he receives from belly dance, he replies, "I like the recognition part. I love the joy and applause of the audience . . . I'm thrilled when I'm out there on stage, and they are excited." Although he does not explicitly talk about belly dance as a form of entertainment, Andy enjoys a great deal of recognition that accompanies being a performer.

Dena, Henry, and Andy primarily define belly dance as entertainment, which does not fit with their understanding of spirituality. Furthermore, it is telling that both Henry and Andy resist constructions of spirituality within belly dance that center on the feminine. These female-focused images do not resonate with male dancers like Henry and Andy, so they protest associating belly dance with a spirituality that they see rooted in the feminine. Some male dancers resist linking belly dance to ancient goddess worship partly because it minimizes the widespread historical custom of male dancers in the Middle East (Karayanni 2009).

Working within belly dance

Crossley (2006a) shows that gym-goers must be able to exercise without thinking about what they are doing in order to become immersed in their workouts. When an activity begins to feel too much like work, letting go and getting lost in the activity can be difficult. Although Agnes is one exception I discussed earlier, instructing students is typically not conducive to many dancers creating spiritual experiences.

Much like performing, teaching others to belly dance is a paid form of work in which a dancer concentrates on an end other than his or her own experience in the dance. Both entertaining an audience and teaching students are activities that are focused on other people. Julia does not infuse belly dance with spiritual meaning when she teaches primarily because she is more focused on her students than herself. When dancers concentrate on other people's experiences, they are less apt to experience spirituality within belly dance. Julia says:

> Especially when I'm teaching, I'm not thinking about myself. I'm thinking about other people ... When I'm planning and dancing through other songs, I'm thinking about what I'm going to do for class ... Half the time I dance is spent thinking about the students and thinking about an upcoming performance and what song is going to be good. . . So, a lot of my dancing is analytical ... Analyzing the music and lesson planning for my students, and a better way to explain something, because student X doesn't understand why, and that type of thing ... When I have to think about dancing, it's obviously not as enjoyable.

Earlier, I discussed how some participants use belly dance as a break away from critical thinking, which helps them experience spirituality within the dance. Here, Julia engages her analytical mind when teaching belly dance, which prevents her from using the dance to take a break from thinking, thereby prohibiting her from experiencing spirituality.

In addition to teaching, some dancers do not experience spirituality when they are focused on correctly executing movements. At the time of our talk, Gwen has been involved in belly dance for about one year. As a relatively new dancer, she is still learning moves, building a movement vocabulary, and focusing on mastering techniques. Especially when she was first learning to belly dance, Gwen reflects, "You're worried about doing the movements and am I going to do these moments right? Is it going to look good? Are people going to like my performance?" However, she has noticed that as time goes on, those concerns "evolve into I'm going to perform for me, and I hope that the audience is going to enjoy it as well."

Presumably, when one is focusing on learning or correctly executing movements, it is difficult for them to get lost in the dance because they concentrate on proper execution. For some dancers, the time spent on the dance and improving one's ability helps people feel more competent, which allows them to focus less on technical execution of movements. Hagedorn (2001) suggests that to some degree competence of the practitioners plays a role in whether a particular dance will take on spiritual meaning.

Whether Nick attaches spirituality to his dance depends on the extent to which he is comfortable with the movements. "Sometimes I'm consciously trying to think how do I do this move or what steps do I do here, particularly when I do the sword dance. I can't always go with the dance. You've got to really think about what you are doing." Nick may be hyper aware of needing to concentrate on his movements, particularly for his sword dances given that he has cut himself when he has dropped the sword. Much like Dena, belly dance is spiritual for Nick "when I'm just doing it for myself."

The relationship between spirituality in belly dance and time is messy. It has been argued that people need to be involved in an art form for some extended length of time to know it well and lose themselves in it (Stewart 2000; Wuthnow 2001). In some ways, this may be true. However, dancers do not create a tangible product, such as a painting or sculpture. They can move to music without necessarily being concerned with the accuracy of those movements. Time may also work against dancers infusing belly dance with spirituality because of other difficulties that come along with being involved in the community for an extended period of time, such as developing negative interpersonal relationships with other dancers. In this way, time can be both a dancer's friend and enemy in regard to spirituality.

Up until this point, I have focused on some very positive aspects of relationships between dancers including support and friendship. However, some participants also navigate tension, ill feelings, and challenging interactions within their dance communities. In Chapter 8, I will devote a great deal of attention to discussing difficult interpersonal relationships between some dancers. Here, I suggest that managing those interactions can feel like "work," thus inhibiting spiritual feelings within belly dance. Shawna, who has been involved in belly dance for over eight years, tells me about dancers who make fun of some other participants' abilities. Shawna says, "The side that is not [spiritual] is the insecure cattiness that comes up with those women that feel that it is a competition . . . I see people in the audience like 'Oh god why is she on stage?' or 'How dare she!' That's when I feel like the spirituality is inhibited," Shawna explains. She continues:

> It's when other people think you shouldn't be on stage unless you're a professional . . . It really just frustrates me . . . I think I just got deeper, and I just saw more of the muck at the bottom . . . because I was on the fringe . . . and everyone was so polite to me, and I was new and shiny and hadn't seen this before. The more I started hanging around groups, and different troupes or individuals or venues, I started seeing this stuff.

Although Shawna initially infused belly dance with spirituality, as her participation in the world continued, she witnessed more cattiness that inhibits infusing belly dance with spiritual meaning. Although her dance technique may improve over time, she has also faced an increasing number of relationship problems with other dancers that inhibit her experiencing spirituality.

"My connection to being spiritual is through Christ"

Participants do not define belly dance as spiritual when their understanding of spirituality is reserved for other activities, such as organized religion. Although Ophelia originally entered belly dance with the intention of the dance serving as her spiritual home, over time, her goals changed. When we meet again, Ophelia has married a man affiliated with a similar religion as the faith in which she was raised. Ophelia wanted to try her husband's religion, so she "switched." Like many other Americans (Stolzenberg *et al.* 1995; Nooney 2006), getting married strengthened Ophelia's commitment to organized religion. Also, Ophelia became more involved in the business aspects of belly dance by teaching classes, instructing workshops, and organizing performances. Ophelia's experiences with spirituality in belly dance greatly changed in the five years in between our two meetings. Ophelia recalls, "When I first started out dancing, I was a little baby." Ophelia was raised Roman Catholic, and at the time she got involved in belly dance, Catholicism "wasn't working out for me." With an artistic background, dance has always been important to Ophelia. Because dance was meaningful to her and she wasn't having positive experiences with organized religion, "I took on belly dance as my spiritual home," Ophelia explains. Ophelia describes experiencing spirituality in belly dance during the beginning of her involvement as "very fulfilling." However, as she got more involved in the business aspects of belly dance, "it kind of erased [spirituality] for me." Ophelia continues:

> You go from being this naïve beginner, and then you see all the dirt behind the curtain. When that happens, it really takes away a page of the loveliness the dance used to be for you. I say shattered your dreams because you're introduced to belly dance, and belly dance is for women, and it's a community, and we're all going to hold hands and sing Kumbayah. That is how we get you in, but it's true. It's presented like that. Then you get in and it's like holy hell it's really complex. Women are complex . . . You start to get to the knitty gritty, and the jealousies and the combativeness comes in . . . I came to the dance for spirituality, and that worked out for a while . . . Gradually [spirituality] just chipped away.

Ophelia's reference to jealousy and competition echoes Shawna's discussion of cattiness. Both of these women highlight an unpleasant side of belly dance that some dancers experience, but generally do not encounter when they first get involved in belly dance. Furthermore, as her participation increased, Ophelia started offering classes and organizing performances. "I can't focus on it being spiritual right now, I've got to get these five people on stage. I got to get a costume change. I got to get tickets at the door," Ophelia explains echoing other dancers' concerns about how belly dance can become work.

Along with getting into the business side of belly dance and experiencing some not so pleasant interactions, Ophelia also married a religious man. "Being married you have that commitment to your spouse," she explains. "It was very important to him that I consider his religion." Ophelia experimented with her new husband's faith and concluded that she liked it. "That has been working out for me . . . That church with him was meeting my [spiritual] needs more than dancing," Ophelia tells me. Given all of the changes both inside and outside of belly dance that Ophelia experienced in the over five years she has been involved in the dance, "belly dancing is nothing what it used to be."

Like Ophelia, other dancers anchor their spirituality in settings other than belly dance. Elsewhere, I discuss how those belly dancers who affiliate with Christianity are less likely to consider belly dance to be spiritual, compared to non-Christians and people of no religious affiliation (Kraus 2009). Some dancers, like Ophelia, have their spiritual needs fulfilled through institutional religious avenues, and they have no desire to construct spiritual meaning within belly dance. These dancers experience spirituality in meditative church experiences.

Similar to Ophelia, Lucy's church meets her spiritual needs. Lucy considers belly dance to be beautiful and captivating, but she does not equate those qualities with spirituality. Lucy comments, "One thing I don't get [from belly dance] is the spiritualness." Although she recognizes that other dancers may experience spirituality within the dance, "I think very much religion is my spirituality and my church." Although she says belly dance is beautiful and "I can be mesmerized, enchanted, and blown away by the power of the dance, I would never call it spiritual." "What, if anything, is spiritual for you?" I wonder. "I am a Baptist girl. I go to church every Sunday, and that is my spiritual fulfillment," Lucy replies. Spirituality, for some dancers like Ophelia and Lucy, is reserved for the religious realm, and these dancers do not define belly dance as religion. Therefore, they do not infuse belly dance with spiritual meaning.

Along with having spiritual needs met through traditional religious institutions, dancers infuse other settings with spiritual meaning. For instance, spirituality does play a role in Jessica's life, but "I don't see [belly dance] as spiritual for me." "How do you define spirituality?" I ask. Jessica replies, "Things that contribute to my spirituality would be music, whether I am performing it or listening to the choir or the organ. Other things would be nature, looking at the beauty of everything. Those are the two that I would most closely express as spirituality." Curious, I ask, "What is different between belly dance music and other music that is spiritual for you?" Jessica responds, "Music has been a part of my life for a whole lot longer. I pursued it with the kind of focus and investment. I thought of getting a diploma in the individual study, and I feel I have a doctorate throughout the years. I am part of an ensemble, and I express my joy in a way I would never do it with dance. That is probably why there is such a close connection there."

Jessica, Ophelia, and Lucy illustrate how some dancers do not define belly dance as spiritual because they reserve their spirituality for activities other than belly dance. Some dancers infuse their other hobbies and interests with spiritual meaning, while some anchor their spirituality in institutionalized religion.

"I'm not a spiritual person"

Although spirituality plays a role in some dancers' lives whether in or outside of belly dance, there is another group of dancers who do not consider themselves to be spiritual at all. Spirituality is not important to them, so they do not infuse any aspects of their lives with spiritual meaning. Leah was raised in a Jehovah's Witness household. But when she turned fourteen, which she refers to as "the age of reason," she and her sister "decided to question why we should even believe if God exists," Leah recalls. Although Leah sometimes finds it challenging to go through life without believing in a higher power, "I don't really see a reason to believe." "How do you define spirituality?" I ask Leah. As someone who was raised outside of the United States, she replies, "That's something I've seen in the U.S., but I don't think that is something you have in [her home country]." When Leah hears people talk about spirituality, she thinks they refer to something that helps them make sense out of life and "makes people want to be good." But, "that's what I think ethics and morals are for. I have really strong ethics that I think comes from my JW teachings . . . I just don't justify it with this ultimate goodness or something. I just think it comes from me. There's nothing out there to make me do it," Leah explains.

Like Leah, Joni does not consider herself a spiritual person. She has never affiliated with a religious organization. Since she does not consider herself a spiritual person, "I don't consider belly dance to be a part of spirituality," Joni tells me. "I guess to some extent it might be, in the fact that it lets you loose and kind of frees you up mentally . . . but I just don't consider myself a spiritual person," Joni continues. "How would you define spirituality?" I ask. Although Joni thinks about spirituality as a "belief in a higher being," echoing Leah's sentiments she does not believe "there is somebody out there guiding my life every day. I think I am responsible for that." Rather than defining belly dance as a potential site for spiritual experiences, Joni uses belly dance as "a mental and physical release to kind of get away from things. I guess if you define being involved in yourself that way as spirituality, then maybe it is, but I have just never seen it that way." Although Joni treats belly dance as a mental escape to "get away from things," this break does not take on spiritual qualities for her unlike many dancers I discussed earlier.

Spiritual reflections

Spirituality in belly dance lies at the intersection of an embodied practice, gender, and interpersonal relationships. The spirituality of belly dance emerges from what people do within the dance. Why and how dancers think about belly dance as spiritual is based on their various experiences within the dance, dancing in different contexts, their definitions of what is spiritual, and their beliefs about the dance.

Dancers experience spirituality when they use the activity to let go and turn off their overactive brains. Different styles, particular steps, and specific movements can take on a ritualistic or meditative quality in ways that facilitate dancers entering "flow" and getting "lost" in the music. At the same time, concentrating on executing movements correctly, entertaining an audience, or teaching students can feel like work by engaging too much of one's thinking mind. Under these circumstances, it is difficult for dancers to take a break from over-analyzing, which hinders their ability to experience flow.

Different contexts and locations support or prevent dancers entering flow. Some dancers are better able to "get into a zone" when they dance alone in their homes and outside distractions are reduced (Kraus 2013). However, some other participants require a group of dancers to create a setting that, for them, feels more communal and ritualistic.

Furthermore, some participants' beliefs support their constructing spirituality within belly dance. How some dancers define the activity complements their understanding of spirituality, while others define the dance in ways that are incompatible with their beliefs (or non-beliefs) about spirituality. For instance, many dancers define belly dance as an art form. Those dancers who associate artistic pursuits with spirituality tend to attach spiritual meaning to belly dance, while others conceptualize spirituality differently and reserve alternative outlets, if any, for spiritual experiences.

Infusing activities with spiritual meaning is one aspect of identity (Magliocco 2004). For some participants, spirituality in belly dance is part of their identity creation. For those dancers who simply do not think of themselves as spiritual people, spirituality is not part of their self-concept. Because they do not associate anything with spirituality, there is no reason for belly dance to be any different. For other dancers, creating spirituality within belly dance is a core part of how they see themselves. In the next chapter, I explore various ways a belly dance identity is both constructed and conferred and how people use additional tools available within belly dance for identity creation.

Chapter 6

A belly dance identity

Ella's Facebook profile picture is a snapshot from when she danced on a Florida beach. While describing the picture to me, Ella recalls moving her fifty-year-old body to the imaginary music in her head. Surrounded by sand and ocean, Ella did not have any musicians accompanying her, so she created her own songs. She recalls a crowd gathering to watch her dance and fondly remembers the compliments she was given about her movements. Despite the fact that she was on vacation states away from her hometown, she spent time belly dancing and broadcasts her dance to anyone who accesses her Facebook page. Not only does this picture capture a fond memory of a beautiful day at the beach, it also announces to everyone who sees it that she belly dances. Of all the various facets of our lives, the important people in it, the things we do, and the places we go, why would someone like Ella choose a picture of herself belly dancing on a beach as her Facebook profile picture? "Because I'm a belly dancer. There ya go," she says.

In contrast, belly dance is only one aspect of Lucy's life. She participates in activities other than belly dance, so "it's not all who I am," Lucy explains. Along with dance, Lucy enjoys watching food programs on television and interacting with cats. "There are people who live and breathe belly dance, and all their friends belly dance, and all they do is think about it," says Lucy. When she has an upcoming show, she devotes a lot of time to the activity by practicing. But after the busyness calms down, Lucy focuses on her other interests. "It's not my entire life. I don't think I can call myself a belly dancer," Lucy explains.

Social worlds and their subcultures exist to the extent that participants identify with the characteristics of that world (Fine 1983). The values and traditions of a group will only influence a person if we identify with that group, recognize the collective norms, and act in ways that fit with group guidelines and expectations (Burke and Stets 2009). As Ella and Lucy illustrate, identification with a subculture varies in the frequency with which people invoke their identity with that group and the centrality or depth of their commitment to it (Fine 2012b).

In this chapter, I explore different degrees to which participants adopt the label of belly dancer and how a variety of indicators marks their level of dedication. In the second part of the chapter, I discuss one specific identifier – the use of stage names – that is relevant within some belly dance subcultures. Particularly, I examine how the creation and adoption of stage names illustrates the processes of role-making and role-taking (Turner 1962).

Who am I? Identities and roles

Identity refers to our internalized sense of who we are in relation to a group (Burke and Stets 2009). Who we are partly depends on the people with whom we interact, the space we occupy, and the scenes in which we are involved (Fine 2012a; Tajfel and Turner 1986). We live in a highly differentiated and complex society. Because people belong to different groups, we have multiple identities based on the various roles we play (Fine 2012b; Merton 1957; Burke and Stets 2009; Stryker and Burke 2000). Ralph Turner (1956:316) defines a role as "a collection of patterns of behavior which are thought to constitute a meaningful unit and deemed appropriate to a person occupying a particular status in society." Statuses can be familial (e.g. mother or brother), occupational (e.g. employee or manager), or social (e.g. Boy Scout or belly dancer). Each of these statuses has norms that accompany them. The extent to which we accept and abide by the expectations is tied to how we identify with any role.

Our identities are arranged in a hierarchical order depending on the degree to which each is meaningful for us and the degree to which we are committed to any particular one (Stryker 1980; Burke and Stets 2009). Some identities are more important for our self-concept than others (Burke and Stets 2009). The more important an identity is for us, the more influential it is for our behavior and the greater role it plays in how we see ourselves. Our most meaningful identities are the ones for which we are more likely to develop skills, talents, and relationships to further support them (Sandstrom et al. 2009).

"I'm a belly dancer. What's your superpower?"

The above question circulates around various belly dance communities, posted on Internet sites and inscribed on T-shirts. Individual dancers who display this phrase on their personal websites and/or clothing claim, and present to the world, the identity of belly dancer. Claiming a particular identity symbolically links people to other members of that social world and those who have been involved in it throughout time (Burke and Stets 2009). Groups and subcultures have symbols, such as jargon and clothing, and the extent to which members adopt these signifiers marks their identification with that culture. There is a meaningful distinction between people who call themselves a belly dancer and those who do not. Participants use several indicators to mark whether they, along with other dancers, identify as a belly dancer.

"Belly dance is a large portion of my life"

Much like other recreational activities, such as running (Altheide and Pfuhl 1980), participants balance the amount of time they devote to dance and their other responsibilities and relationships. For people who call themselves belly dancers, the activity takes up much of their time. It is not an activity in which they occasionally dabble and then forget about until their next lesson. Rather they spend a great deal of time thinking about belly dance, practicing, and studying their music. "Belly dance is a large portion of my life," Alexandra begins. "It's not something that is just an hour a week," Alexandra adds as she contrasts her deeper level of involvement in the dance with people who only take a weekly class. "When I'm not dancing, I'm thinking about it. I read Arabic just to understand the song and the culture that I'm performing," Alexandra continues. Belly dance is a large part of Alexandra's life because she spends a great deal of time engaged in activities related to it. "It's an important part of my identity," Alexandra says. "If people ask me how I spend my time or what I do, I would tell them I'm a professor, but part of what I do, part of who I am is a belly dancer," she explains. How dancers like Alexandra incorporate their dance identity indicates psychological centrality, or how important an identity is in the way one thinks about herself (Stryker and Serpe 1994).

As opposed to Alexandra, "I feel like I am someone who belly dances," Candie tells me. Contrasting her peripheral involvement with some of her friends who identify as belly dancers, Candie remarks, "It's just a different commitment level, and I would rather it be fun than an obligation." "Did it ever feel like it was an obligation?" I ask. "Definitely," she succinctly replies. "I felt like I was letting [her dance group] down a lot because I wasn't able to be as committed as they were," Candie says. Since having children, Candie's involvement in belly dance diminished. "When you were more committed did you feel like you were a person who belly dances or a belly dancer?" "I would say earlier, I would have identified myself as a belly dancer, but I think the more people I see, I realize there is so much I don't know. How could I call myself a belly dancer when these women dedicate so much time and effort to this platform?" Candie responds. That Candie feels like her lack of involvement might disappoint her group suggests that there is a level of participation typically required of her, and when she can't meet those expectations, her troupe mates may look down on her. Candie and Alexandra suggest that a belly dancer identity best fits participants with greater commitments to the activity who spend more hours involved in it. Identity theory suggests that those identities to which people have the greatest commitment will rank near the top of an identity hierarchy (Stryker and Burke 2000). Alexandra, who is highly committed to belly dance, incorporates belly dance into her identity, while Candie who has less time to devote to it, refrains from thinking of herself as a belly dancer.

"It's a lifestyle"

When a leisure pursuit becomes a regular part of people's normal routine and they become immersed in it, their identification with the activity becomes salient beyond a hobby (Altheide and Pfuhl 1980). Belly dance infiltrates multiple areas of several dancers' lives, suggesting that their participation is more diffused than something in which they occasionally participate.

"To me, it's a lifestyle," Mark tells me after four years of involvement in the dance. Belly dance is a large and salient part of his identity. Identity salience refers to the likelihood of the identity being acted in a particular situation. The higher an identity ranks in our hierarchy, the greater the likelihood that the identity will be invoked in any particular situation (Stryker and Serpe 1994). "I'll go out shopping somewhere, and I'll see a scarf and think I can use that for a costume. My brain goes straight to belly dance and how I can apply stuff. I'll hear a song on the radio, and I'll think that would be great to do a choreography to that." Mark is among many dancers who label themselves as belly dancers because they adopt belly dance as a central component of who they are as people, and thus, invoke a belly dance identity in various situations. Dancers like Mark see clothing that they think would be good for costumes, and they hear songs outside of a dance context to which they imagine a choreography.

However, dancers who do not claim a belly dancer identity tend to isolate their participation in belly dance. "I don't really even incorporate belly dance into my identity at all. It's just something that I do," Scarlett tells me. About being a person who belly dances rather than a belly dancer, Scarlett continues, "It's sort of a tangential part of my life, especially right now. Even when it was a big part of my life, I still wouldn't say I was a belly dancer. Even back then because I was still learning. But also because . . . I think performing for money or at events is a big part of that, to take that title, and it's not something I do." Scarlett reiterates that belly dance is a not a core part of how she sees herself. She believes that performing, especially for pay, is a norm that accompanies the role of belly dancer. Along with belly dance playing a tangential role in her life, she does not adhere to an expectation that a belly dancer performs. Therefore, she does not claim a belly dancer identity.

"A belly dancer is a professional performer"

Dancers who think of themselves as beginners or intermediates and amateurs generally do not claim a belly dance identity. Those dancers who adopt a belly dance identity consider themselves to be advanced and semi-professional or professional dancers (although the vast majority of them do not make a living with belly dance). These dancers construct their participation in belly dancer as deeper and more intense compared to some dancers for whom belly dance is a mere hobby. People who perceive their involvement as "professional" treat belly dance more seriously with a heightened sense of responsibility and commitment.

For many participants, performing is a catalyst for identifying themselves as belly dancers. In the summer of 2014, I participate in multiple public performances with my troupe and dance at several drum circles. My involvement in belly dance greatly increases during this summer. One night I converse with my husband about how belly dance has recently become more important to me. Given that I have not remembered belly dance being so personally meaningful, I am surprised by how much I enjoy participating in the community. "Rachel, I think this summer has been a turning point for you," my husband remarks about how often I have been dancing. A turning point refers to the feeling that I am not the same person that I used to be. It is a crucial experience that greatly alters one's path and may signal the beginning of a new direction. Turning points typically occur when someone re-evaluates his or her identity (Strauss 1959). During this summer, I perform more, which is a more public spectacle than dancing privately at home or in a classroom. Due to the public nature of performing, I am aware that I will be scrutinized, which motivates me to rehearse more often than when I'm not scheduled to perform. Furthermore, I focus on polishing my movements and cues because (1) as an American Tribal Style dancer, the other dancers can better follow my lead when I give clear cues and (2) I don't want to disappoint the other dancers in my group by being a weak dancer. All of these changes mark a "new direction" for me.

"I am a belly dancer, because first of all, I am a professional belly dancer," Rose tells me after pursuing the activity for almost ten years. "That's why I would call myself a belly dancer as opposed to somebody who belly dances. I feel that I take it seriously, and that when somebody approaches me that either knows that I dance, or when I'm in costume, I feel like it's my obligation to give them knowledge [about belly dance]," Rose continues. Rose claims a belly dance identity partly because she feels she is familiar enough with belly dance to educate others. To Rose, a professional is not someone who earns their living at belly dance, in fact she does not even mention money. Rather, according to Rose, someone who is "serious" about the activity, is knowledgeable, and has a responsibility (expectation) to educate other people characterizes a belly dance professional. By feeling responsible to educate non-dancers, Rose suggests that belly dance is something that either people do not know much about or do not have a level of understanding about the activity that some belly dancers would like them to have. As a self-identified professional, Rose wants to help make the public more aware of how she, and other members of the belly dance community, believes the activity should be viewed.

In addition to performing and feeling responsible to educate outsiders, teaching also factors into whether and when someone claims a belly dance identity. Arlene has participated in belly dance for over thirty-five years. "The first couple of years when I was taking classes" Arlene thought of herself as someone who belly dances. Arlene began to consider herself a belly dancer when she started teaching. "You have to have that level of confidence," the seasoned dancer in her sixties explains. Both teaching and performing signal a level of security and courage that many participants associate with a belly dancer identity, but not all dancers develop that feeling of comfort.

Unlike Rose and Arlene, Gemma was involved in belly dance for less than two years. "I would have been happy if I had said I know how to belly dance or I know something about belly dancing, but I never would have said that I was a belly dancer," Gemma reflects on her identity when she was actively involved in belly dance. Her few performances were at very small events and she generally felt they did not go well. Gemma typically was not comfortable feeling "exposed" while performing, and she remembers some mistakes made during the shows. "A belly dancer is a professional performer," Gemma says. During her involvement in belly dance, Gemma "didn't feel like I was at that level of skill." Her perceived lack of talent prohibits Gemma from thinking of herself as a professional, and therefore, a belly dancer. Performing and teaching suggest that one is more immersed in the activity compared to those who attend an occasional class. They also suggest a level of commitment to practicing and talent.

"I've done the work to learn the culture"

People are involved in leisure activities to different degrees, and their skill levels vary. How often and with whom someone trains marks the identity of a belly dancer. Henry studied ballet for a year in high school, learned English country dancing, and dabbled in line dance. However, these experiences are in his background more than a part of how he identifies himself, suggesting that they do not rank high on his identity hierarchy. "I'm a belly dancer. That is my training," Henry tells me. Like many other dancers, Henry's dance lineage influences identifying himself as a belly dancer. Henry has taken multiple classes with teachers who have studied with Suhalia Salimpour, the daughter of Jamila whom many people credit with the founding of modern belly dance in America. Henry has also taken classes with people who have been trained by Carolena Nericcio who is credited with codifying the American Tribal Style of belly dance. Furthermore, Henry has taken classes with some of the most popular and sought-after tribal fusion dancers, such as Rachel Brice and Zoe Jakes. His connection to many of the great dancers and his years of training are "why I feel like I can say I'm a belly dancer. I've done the work to learn the culture and learn the styling to develop my voice inside that style." Henry extends the importance of his dance training by suggesting that not only has he studied with some of the very best dancers in the country, he has studied long enough to develop his own style based on his training. "Regardless of what my other [dance] influences may be, my core vocabulary is belly dance," Henry concludes.

Unlike Henry, some other dancers do not feel they have the knowledge or training to call themselves belly dancers. Although she has been involved in the activity for over twenty-five years, Jessica contrasts her experiences as a self-proclaimed belly dance amateur with her more professional experiences as a musician. "I've never done the things that, to me, would indicate I am a professional [belly dancer]," Jessica begins. Although she takes belly dance classes, Jessica has not "studied with the best of the best, like with my music," she tells me. Unlike Henry, Jessica has not taken classes with some of the most accomplished and popular belly dance instructors. Furthermore, she has not taken many belly dance workshops, attended seminars, or studied in other countries. She also does not "read the belly dance literature" and she does not belong to any national organizations. Contrasting her peripheral participation in belly dance with her deep commitment to music, Jessica continues, "With music, I belong to different groups . . . I am a part of all that, studying with the top people . . . there is the difference." Along with not acquiring a level of ability and knowledge that more professional dancers have, Jessica hints at the time discrepancy between her involvement in music and her participation in belly dance. Clearly, Jessica's involvement in music ranks higher than belly dance on her identity hierarchy. Jessica and Henry demonstrate that the amount and type of training that people invest in the activity are expectations that factor into whether someone claims a belly dance identity.

"Costuming is a big part of a troupe look"

Clothing is an important resource that communicates group membership to subcultural insiders and outsiders (Wilkins 2008). Whereas fashion can illustrate belonging, it can also divide members based on their adherence to and adoption of an approved wardrobe (Wilkins 2008). Along with thinking of oneself as a professional with a relatively deep commitment to learning all about the activity, one additional marker of a belly dance identity is one's costume collection. Teachers and troupe directors make assumptions about participants' dance identities using similar markers as dancers themselves. In addition, instructors gauge commitment levels of their students partly by observing their acquisition of costumes. About when her students are ready to participate in her professional troupe, Naomi, an instructor and troupe director of many years comments, "I'm looking at how reliable and committed someone is, and if they're open to constructive criticism, general positive attitude/friendliness, and how their technique progresses. I look for whether someone is actively expanding their costume collection." "Are these all markers of a dance identity?" I ask. Naomi replies about the additional importance of costumes:

> When I look for someone who is pro troupe material, I do need to see a multifaceted engagement . . . I don't think investing in costume pieces over time is necessarily the only or the most important marker of a dancer identity that exists. But, since so much of running a dance troupe is about how we present ourselves to the public, I want my dancers' visual presentation to be in line with the image we're trying to present. So, while I'm all about encouraging my dancers to work on the obvious facets of their dance identity that go along with performing – stage presence and technique – I don't want to neglect the costuming portion.

The acquisition of costumes is interpreted as both a literal and figurative investment. Expanding one's costume collection is an investment of time and money. At the same time, those costumes signify to dancers like Naomi, how much the dancer is invested in the activity. So dancers assume that people with large or at least growing costume collections demonstrate a deeper commitment level to belly dance compared to people with relatively smaller collections who are not seeking to add more to their dance "stash."

How we see ourselves is rooted in how other people respond to us (Burke and Stets 2009). In this way, identity is conferred by other people in addition to being claimed. Not only do participants consider whether they identify as belly dancers, instructors and troupe leaders also make judgments which influence self-assessments. Building one's belly dance wardrobe is one expectation associated with the role of belly dancer, and the extent to which one adheres to this norm influences how a student and instructor evaluates his or her identity as a belly dancer.

"Unfortunately, costuming is a big part of the troupe look," Dena comments. "I was looking at my costume *closets* [emphasizing the plural of closet] the other day, thinking about what I should keep and what I should let go.

Of course, there's always another costume idea percolating in my brain," Dena says. She continues, "I know few dancers who have been at this for a while who are not dedicated costume collectors." Dena suggests that people who have been involved in belly dance for a long time acquire several costumes and accessories, while people who remain on the edges of the community do not have an extensive belly dance wardrobe.

Ability, knowledge, performing, commitment, integration, and costuming are markers that participants use to adopt, and in some cases confer, a dancer identity. Those dancers who feel particularly skilled and dedicate much time and resources to belly dance are more likely to think of themselves and other participants as belly dancers. Dancers who judge their abilities as less advanced and feel less committed to the activity tend to avoid the label of belly dancer. Within some dance communities, adopting a dance name (or not) also marks a belly dance identity with a style or group. How dance names are chosen and what those names represent illustrates how some dancers construct their identity within various constraints surrounding the role of belly dancer.

Adopting a stage name

Names act as symbols, represent people, and convey meanings about them. We act toward objects and labels, including names, based on the meanings they have been assigned (Blumer 1969; Burke and Stets 2009; Strauss 1959). When a person self-selects a name, the identifier serves as a mini description by revealing information about a person that she or he wants to share with others. For instance, in online environments people use screen names to communicate ideas and images. Users associate themselves with particular characteristics based on their screen name, and the name becomes a prominent identifier of who they are, their interests, and what they want from their online interactions (Waskul 2003).

When we choose names for ourselves, we opt for identifiers that we think will solicit positive reactions from people, while avoiding those names that we think may invite a negative response. The meanings associated with names will depend on certain audiences and contexts. What is considered positive or negative will vary depending on the situation in which the name is used. These goals of seeking positive feedback, while avoiding negative reactions mirror Goffman's (1967) concept of defensive face-work. By face-work, Goffman refers to the actions we take to be consistent with positive impressions people have of us. Maintaining face is associated with decency and social acceptability (Scott 2010). Strategies to "save face" help meet our "face needs" (Brown and Levinson 1987), such as gaining acceptance and approval from others. Face-work serves to counteract incidents that might threaten affirmative ways people view us.

Role-making, role-taking, and stage names

Role-making refers to how individuals create their roles using behaviors, gestures, and appearance. While roles are constrained by norms from the communities in which they are situated, people modify and redefine roles to suit their needs and preferences (Turner 1962). Within any given role, we have a certain amount of flexibility to assert our creativity. At the same time, there are limits placed on our freedom to enact our roles. For instance, as a college professor, I have leeway in the reading I assign my students, assessment methods, classroom activities, and how I present information. However, it's probably not a good idea for me to use a lot of profanity when interacting with students regardless of how much I may feel like cussing in front of my class. I am restrained partly by my university standards, but also by my own desire not to curse. Therefore, some of these restraints are self-imposed, while some are rooted in our relationships with other people and the communities to which we belong.

In this section, I discuss stage naming practices. Whether and how belly dancers choose dance names reveals something about how dancers see themselves and how they want to present themselves to the world given the constraints of the belly dance communities in which they are situated. Dancers select names that are personally meaningful to them (self-imposed guidelines) and which fit within accepted community standards (cultural norms), while avoiding names that may lead to others perceiving them in negative ways (interpersonal constraints). Therefore, naming practices illustrate expectations dancers experience both inside and outside the belly dance community.

People belonging to different groups strategically create names to identify themselves as members of those social worlds (Williams 2006). Similarly, the adoption of names varies depending on which style of belly dance one participates in and the specific idioculture of one's group. For instance, I have been a part of three performance troupes. I used a stage name with my first two groups. My first group performed mostly cabaret/nightclub styles of belly dance, which are some of the styles most closely related to traditional Middle Eastern and North African dance. Selecting dance names, particularly Middle Eastern names, further maintains those cultural roots. My second troupe danced improvisational tribal style (ITS), which is an offshoot of ATS. Although using stage names is less common in ATS and ITS given that they are farther removed from Middle Eastern and North African cultures, most of the members in my ITS group used a stage name. I continued using a name as dictated by my group's idioculture. The third troupe with whom I currently dance is an official ATS group. No one in my troupe uses a dance name when performing with our troupe, most likely because ATS is an American codified dance. Similar to following the idioculture of my ITS group, I dropped my dance name after joining my ATS troupe.

For various reasons, some participants do not use dance names. Like my experiences, some dancers do not affiliate with groups or perform styles in which adopting a dance name is common. Liz is more involved in the tribal fusion style of belly dance than the traditional Egyptian or cabaret styles of dance. Much like ATS and ITS, tribal fusion is a hybrid dance form and less rooted in Middle Eastern and North African dance. Therefore, cultural norms within cabaret style belly dance communities are less applicable to tribal fusion dance. "It's another reason why I think choosing a dance name is silly," Liz begins. "It's not Middle Eastern anymore. It's got its own identity in America." Furthermore, as a light-skinned woman with light-colored hair, Liz says she is "not Middle Eastern and can't even pretend to be. I am quite obviously not." Liz does not think that using a Middle Eastern name would be believable because her appearance is far removed from how she imagines the appearance of people with Middle Eastern and North African roots. In addition, Liz "likes my name. It really encompasses me and my personality." Liz attempted to choose a dance name, but "I end up not liking it and not feeling like it represents me." Liz wants a name that portrays how she sees herself, and adopting a Middle Eastern or North African dance name does not meet that goal.

Like Liz, Macy researched Arabic names but couldn't find the "word I am looking for." In her sixties, Macy wanted an Arabic name that reflected a grandmother, because "I am a grandmother . . . and it lets people remember that I am old enough that I can't do some of the things these younger [dancers] do." In her earlier dance experiences, Macy would drop to her knees and execute movements primarily on bended knees or lying on the stage. However, as she aged, she developed difficulties with her joints. Therefore, she no longer performs floor work, and she wants her audience to understand her physical limitations. Because she could not find a name that "feels right" and reflects her stage in life and dance capabilities, Macy ultimately decided not to adopt a dance name. Both Macy and Liz wanted names that matched how they see themselves and how they want others to view them. In both of their cases, choosing a name would not allow them to remain consistent with their self-perceptions (self-imposed restraint) and how they want other people to see them (cultural and interpersonal restraints). Furthermore, these two dancers do not belong to groups with idiocultures that encourage the adoption of a dance name. Therefore, they elect not to adopt dance names. Although Liz and Macy do not use dance names, other dancers do select a stage name. These participants use several strategies to choose names that are, to varying degrees, reflective of how they see themselves.

"I wanted to integrate who I am into belly dance"

Like online users who adopt screen names that are close to their first names (Waskul 2003), some belly dancers choose names that are similar to their birth names. For instance, Rukan chose her name partly because her birth name also starts with an "R.""I wanted to integrate who I am into belly dancing," Rukan says. Belly dance is also a way for Rukan to experience personal and spiritual growth, so she wanted her name "to represent who I am. Like basically what you see is what you get." Choosing a dance name that is similar to her birth name allows Rukan to both participate in the customs of her dance style and maintain ties to how she views herself.

Second, some dancers choose names that reflect a fantasy version of how they see themselves. Their dance name rarely symbolizes an entirely different identity. Selecting names that are extensions of how they view themselves is similar to role-playing gamers and people in Second Life who create characters that resemble how they view themselves outside of their online or gaming worlds (Fine 2002; Waskul and Lust 2004; Waskul and Martin 2010). Furthermore, in her research on relationships between customers and dancers at a high end gentlemen's club, Frank (1988) demonstrates that to varying degrees, club performers choose stage characters that, at least in part, reflect some aspect of themselves.

Some belly dancers select names that reflect their hobbies and interests outside of belly dance, which illustrates their desire to at least partly combine their dance persona with everyday selves. When she first selected a stage name, Naia Al'Abbasi spent "months and months of researching.""I know in dancing you are not necessarily stuck with that name the rest of your life, but it is still an important decision, and you want something that reflects you and your personality," Naia explains. "I get compared to water a lot when I dance," she says. Naia's name is a shortened version of the Greek word Naiad, which refers to water nymphs in Greek mythology. Al'Abbasi was a name she inherited from her troupe leader at the time as it is somewhat customary within some cabaret style communities for students to adopt the name of their teachers. "All of her top students had the last name Al'Abbasi," Naia explains. However, since that time, Naia formed her own troupe. "It felt false to have the last name Al'Abbasi since I was no longer part of her troupe. I was a leader now and needed my own last name to pass on to my students," Naia says. "I chose Abal similar to the way I chose Naia. I searched Arabic name sites until I found something that I both liked the sound of and the meaning. Abal is Arabic for wild rose," Naia tells me. Naia now uses Naia Abal. The name Naia originally used was no longer meaningful to her after she left her first troupe. Similar to some Pagans who change their names as they move through different stages of participation in their communities (Magliocco 2004), changing belly dance names illustrates how the use of names is fluid.

"What do you like about the meaning wild rose?" I inquire. "It had nothing to do with belly dance, but is more about how I felt with my marital divorce," Naia begins. She tells me about a song called "Where the Wild Roses Grow" by Nick Cave. This song is "very depressing and chilling," Naia explains. Naia used to listen to Nick Cave's music with her first husband "and this is one of the songs that really stood out to me when he introduced me to this artist," Naia remembers. "The song is a murder ballad where the guy courts a girl they call the wild rose and kills her," she explains. "I just identified with the wild rose," Naia tells me. "Dancing to this song was one of the most therapeutic experiences of my life," Naia states. No doubt a divorce can be complicated and traumatic. When her original last name was no longer significant to her, Naia chose another deeply meaningful name symbolizing a fond memory of great healing.

"Ha as in haha, and Kan as in khaaaaaaaan," the dancer exclaims while scooting to the edge of his chair, sitting straight up, and raising his fist in the air. "Like the wrath of Kahn," he continues. Hakan chose his name many years ago when he started dancing with a Turkish band that performed in bars. One of the band members, a friend of Hakan's, wanted to display a poster with the band's name and his name as their featured dancer. "I will have these posters in three weeks, and there is no way I am going to put my band featuring a dancer with a generic European name. The dancer name I'm going to put up is Zoltan if you don't choose a dancer name," Hakan recalls his friend saying to him. So even though Hakan "loved this particular person, she was not going to be the one to choose my dancer name." He found Hakan in an English/Turkish dictionary, did some research, and learned that it is a very common Turkish name. "The word means sultan or king," he tells me. Hakan considers himself "a very theatrical person." He calls himself "light-hearted," so the first part of his name (Ha) "is very indicative of my personality." "I'm also, to be gentle, a geek, so being able to reference *Star Trek* or *Star Wars* or having Batman as part of a character are things I appreciate being able to do," Hakan explains about the second part of his name. Indeed, Hakan is well known in some belly dance circles for dressing up as Batman for various belly dance performances. Furthermore, referencing a king or a sultan is highly gendered. Hakan likes to showcase his masculinity in dance, so it is fitting that his name embodies masculinity. In addition, Hakan wanted to find a name that he thought would enhance his credibility of being associated with a Turkish band. In this way, his selection of a name was constrained by community standards. He couldn't be "Bob the belly dancer" because that name would not fit within the setting of a Turkish musical group because Bob is not a common Turkish name. Within the norms of the context, the name "Bob" isn't believable. If the group wants to be taken seriously as a Turkish band, they need a dancer with a legitimate name that fits within the boundaries of their community. Therefore, within community constraints of finding a Turkish name, Hakan chose a name that reflects his personality, his interests outside of dance, and his identity as a male dancer.

"I do a lot of Turkish dancing, so I have a Turkish name"

A third technique some dancers use to select names that are meaningful to them is to choose identifiers that represent their dance style. Electra was no stranger to performing other forms of dance and in theater productions before she got involved in belly dance. "I felt like I was shining," the dancer says of her performing. "I felt alive, and it had been a long time since I had been on stage. I had always loved to be a performer," Electra says. Electra danced with a primarily cabaret/nightclub style group and her group's idioculture encouraged the use of stage names. Although Electra did not select a name with Middle Eastern or North African origins, she chose a name that reflects how she feels when she dances. Like Hakan, the process of Electra selecting her name illustrates adherence to her group's norms and the personal creativity of role-making with the self-imposed constraints of wanting a name that is meaningful to her.

Similar to Electra, Izmaragd chose a name that reflects her Turkish style of belly dance. Izmaragd is Russian for emerald, according to the dancer. She believes the name also sounds Turkish, so she thought, "that would work." "Is it good that it sounds Turkish?" I ask. "I do a lot of Turkish dancing, so having a Turkish name" fits with her style of dancing. Furthermore, her name "also works for the SCA [Society for Creative Anachronism] because it's a documentable name. It actually existed in the time period," Izmaragd tells me. Because she is fairly active in both belly dance circles and the SCA, the dancer wanted a name that she could use for both communities. Therefore, Izmaragd's name is shaped by the culture of her belly dance community and by her participation in the SCA that dictates participants have documentable (authentic for the time period and location) names.

"In remembrance of her and my friendship"

Similar to some Pagans who choose a name to match their lineage to a particular ethnic culture (Magliocco 2004), a belly dance name can signify one's cultural roots. Gabi's name has changed slightly over the more than fifteen years that she has been involved in dance. Early on in her dance experiences, Gabi was short for Gabriela. However, now in her thirties, Gabi wants to link herself to her Greek ancestry. "I wanted something more closely related to

Greek, because I'm from the Greek people," Gabi explains. Since then, Gabi has changed her name to Gabrielia. Like we have seen with other dancers, Gabi's decision to alter her name is a mix of cultural guidelines and her desire to have a name that links her to ethnic roots.

Along with choosing names that connect a dancer to his or her heritage, several dancers select a name that honors meaningful people in their lives. Rania's stage name is based on the youngest daughter of a Saudi man with whom she was friends in college. "She is just a charming little girl, a born performer," Rania says. The dancer chose her name "in remembrance of [the daughter] and my friendship with this colleague and that wonderful summer that we were able to spend together," Rania explains. Her connection to this family clearly has had a lasting, powerful effect on Rania. "My friendship with this person caused me to become very interested in Middle Eastern culture, and that's probably what led to my desire to experience that culture through dance," Rania explains. Adopting a dance name that represents this family honors Rania's friendship with them and their influence on her pursuing belly dance.

"I want a name that is respectable"

Much like people with an online presence who avoid names with negative connotations (Waskul 2003), many belly dancers attempt to avoid names that elicit undesirable images. The meanings of symbols, such as names, are guided by and shared within a culture. They are also arbitrary and can differ across contexts (Burke and Stets 2009). Because some belly dance names, particularly those used by cabaret and nightclub style dancers, are typically rooted in the Middle East and surrounding areas, fully understanding a name's traditional meaning can be difficult. It can be challenging for dancers to find names that are meaningful for them while considering whether the name they select represents something undesirable in its host culture. Also, the pronunciation of foreign names can be challenging to some Western audiences. Some dancers want to be sure that Americans can correctly pronounce the names they choose to avoid an unflattering mispronunciation and by extension, unfavorable impressions of themselves.

Shuvani, who has been dancing for close to forty years, first used the name Marika el Khadira, which was "the closest to [her birth name] I could come up with." However, people typically pronounced her name as a Spanish slang word for "slut, but I think the actual meaning has something to do with swine," Shuvani tells me. "It's a Hungarian name, pronounced MAH rah kah, but it usually got pronounced Ma REE kah," she tells me. "Too bad because I really liked that name." "So after about a year I just dropped the stage name and danced under [her birth name]." Even though Shuvani liked her original dance name, she decided not to use it because of unfavorable interactions with some audience members and she did not want to be associated with a negative image. Nowadays, Shuvani uses her birth name and/or Shuvani, which translates to "wise woman." Given that she is almost seventy years old, the meaning of her name seems fitting because wisdom is something we ideally gain as we age.

Wanting to avoid a name with a negative connotation is a common concern among dancers. Asena believes that belly dancers already have a "questionable" reputation among some segments of the American population. She asked some of her Turkish friends to help her choose a name. "I was telling them I want a name that is respectable," Asena recalls. One of her friends told her about a belly dancer in Turkey who was very well known and highly respected, "which in Turkey is not that common," Asena says. "Belly dancers are very iffy characters. That's why he gave me that name." Because Asena believes that belly dancers are ill-perceived in many cultures, she did not want to contribute to a problematic reputation by choosing a derogatory name. Like many other dancers who use stage names, both Shuvani and Asena were part of groups with idiocultures that encouraged the adoption of a dance name. However, how both women chose their names was shaped by larger cultural constraints of not wanting to be associated with something negative and, in Shuvani's case, interpersonal concerns of mispronunciation.

"I like the way that one sounded"

Rather than focusing on the meaning of a name, some participants select a dance name based on aesthetics. Although Amara Hazine's dance name refers to an attractive gem, she did not choose her name for the meaning. Rather, "I picked it because I really like the name," she tells me. Also, there is a fairly well-known belly dancer in another state who uses Amara. To distinguish herself from this other dancer, Amara added Hazine. "I thought it sounded really beautiful. The two of them together I just thought it flowed really well," Amara explains.

Along with the women, a few of the male dancers with whom I spoke also chose names (when they use names other than their birth names) based on how the name sounds. To Valizan's knowledge, his name doesn't have a particular meaning. The dancer discovered it while reading an article that mentioned a world-renowned trumpet player from the 1950s named Louis Valizan. "I thought it was a very exciting and unique kind of name," Valizan tells me. The dancer doesn't have a special affinity for jazz music or any background in playing the trumpet, he just "loved the last name." "When I started dancing

I was in a medieval re-enactment group where you had to take on a different persona, and I started off with a different name,"Valizan tells me. "What name were you using?" I ask. "Jeremy Keith of Rose Petal Pond," he exclaims as we both burst out laughing. We have a mutual understanding that this name would not be believable or appropriate within a context rooted in Middle Eastern and North African culture. "It's a very English name, and I was playing an English persona,"Valizan explains. However, he didn't like that name. "It was boring, and I decided I wanted an Arabic persona, and I liked Valizan better." In addition to liking the sound of his name, similar to other dancers, Valizan's name selection was shaped, in part, by the community standards in which he operates. Although his American Tribal Style group does not encourage stage names, many people in belly dance circles met Valizan through this re-enactment group (there is a great deal of overlap between participation in belly dance and this group). Because he was already known as Valizan, he decided to continue using it as his dance name.

"I was so flattered by her comment"

Role-taking reflects our desire to present ourselves in ways that conform to other people's perceptions of us (Turner 1956, 1962). Some dancers adopt names that other people give them because they like the sound and/or meaning of the name, mirroring role-making strategies. Furthermore, they do not view the suggested names as problematic or potentially derogatory, such as having a negative meaning in its country of origin or prone to mispronunciation. Zhenna received her name when she was dancing at a belly dance convention with her troupe at the time. "An Iraqi dancer from Canada told me at dinner that my dance name should be Zhenna because it means heavenly. She said I had a heavenly smile. I was so flattered by her comment that I asked her to spell it and have used it ever since." Zhenna says the event was "a highlight for me." "I've taken several workshops with [the dancer from Canada] since that time and she still remembers me," Zhenna explains.

Similar to Zhenna, Dunya Alamira was given her name by the owner of a Greek establishment at which she danced during her first solo performance in a restaurant. The owner "knew that I was trying to find a name," Dunya tells me. The dancer in her forties remembers the owner saying to her, "You're so full of life!" "I was just so excited to be there dancing," Dunya tells me. At some point in the evening, the restaurant owner exclaimed, "Dunya Alamira!" "What does that mean?" she inquired. When the owner told her that the name meant "princess of light," Dunya thought, "Oh a princess! OK!" When I ask Dunya why she liked having the word princess in her name, she responds, "Because I like the cabaret style. I like the shiny. I like the bling, and it just makes me think of all the jewels," Dunya smiles. Both Zhenna and Dunya Alamira considered the suggested names flattering and attractive. Although other people originally suggested their respective names, these dancers contemplated the extent to which they felt the name "fit" how they view themselves, similar to some role-making strategies.

A role–person merger

Identification with groups and the adoption of their idiocultures is a matter of degree. People have varying levels of commitment to the groups in which they participate (Fine 2012b). Selimah, a dancer now in her forties, has used her belly dance name since "the very beginning when I was like sixteen years old," she tells me. In fact, "I can claim it as my name, legally. Because it's been such a part of me for so many years, I've thought about adding it to my name legally on paper," Selimah says. Changing her legal name to her belly dance name is a profound example of what Ralph Turner (1978) calls a "role–person merger" in which a person ceases to compartmentalize roles.

Those participants for whom belly dance is a livelihood spend a great deal of their lives engaged in activities that revolve around belly dance. For instance, Ruby, now in her fifties, has been involved in the dance for almost thirty years and earns her living through belly dance. At the time of our last talk, Ruby made all of her money through belly dance related activities although she had other sources of income when she first became involved in belly dance. Some time ago, Ruby legally changed her name from her birth name to her dance name. "I do business as Ruby Jazayre, and my business is listed as Ruby Jazayre, so I can cash checks as Ruby Jazayre," she tells me. "Now I'm teaching [at the collegiate level], in theater and dance, and teaching belly dancers. I have a troupe, and then I have my traveling troupe." In Ruby's case, belly dance is such a large part of her existence, the role of belly dancer becomes a prominent part of her identity, which is reflected in her legal name change.

Role mergers also occur when the attitudes and behaviors associated with a role are carried over into other situations that don't immediately call for that role. For instance, many role playing gamers don't leave their names at the end of the game (Fine 2002). Gamers may identify themselves to others outside of a game by their game name, such as signing documents or letters with their character's name (Fine 2002). Some belly dancers' names are such an integrated part of their identity that they are known by their names across different contexts. Although they may not legally change their names, their dance name becomes their primary identifier in and out of belly dance circles. The extent to which and how frequently people identify someone with a role increases the likelihood that the person will merge that role with their person (Turner 1978). Most of Gabi's friends are belly dancers or involved in the SCA, and many of these people call her Gabi rather than use her birth name. Although her family and people at work primarily know her by her birth name, some of her friends outside of belly dance know her as Gabi. Just like some Pagans who are known mostly by their Pagan names both inside and outside of their communities (Magliocco 2004), dancers like Gabi are known primarily by their belly dance names even when they are not in a belly dance context. In this sense, Gabi's identity as a belly dancer is not temporarily suspended when she participates in other areas of her life. In fact, her now husband didn't know her birth name until three months after they met and she "met his kids as Gabi too," she tells me. Continuing to use their name suggests that dancers like Gabi have identities that remain constant across different settings and situations (Burke and Stets 2009).

Revisiting identity

Belly dance is an activity that people experience along a continuum. On one end of the spectrum are participants who are aware of and adhere to a variety of general community norms, such as dedicating time to develop a certain level of ability, commitment to one's group, gaining knowledge, seeking out good instructors, and building a respectable costume collection. These norms, amongst others, are the basis for owning and conferring the identity of belly dancer. On the other end, are people who do not devote much of their time and energy to practicing or performing belly dance. Participants who are not heavily involved in belly dance have other interests and responsibilities that require their attention. Because these less involved dancers do not closely adhere to the norms associated with the role of belly dancer most of the time, they hesitate to claim the identity of belly dancer. These two ends of the continuum mirror the distinction between a hobby and a career. Those for whom belly dance is a hobby experience the dance more as an "activity enclave" (Cohen and Taylor 1992) that is one among many roles they play. Conversely, those for whom belly dance is closer to a career (regardless of whether they make a living through belly dance) view belly dance as one of their primary roles. For these dancers, belly dance is more central to their sense of self and diffused throughout their life.

The specific practice of selecting a dance name (or not) also signifies identification with different belly dance styles and particular groups. Like many other roles, belly dancers are both constrained by a variety of factors when selecting a dance name and creatively work within these guidelines. To varying degrees, norms within different styles of dance shape whether dancers adopt names, and if so, the names dancers select. At the same time, participants work within self-imposed constraints to adopt names that are symbolic and personally meaningful to them. Furthermore, not wanting to be viewed unfavorably, dancers work to avoid names that can be mispronounced (in negative ways) and/or have derogatory meanings. Therefore, rather than serving as a completely alternative identifier, most dancers incorporate aspects of their everyday experiences into their dance name. Dancers want to identify with the name they select. In order to achieve identification, they borrow from other aspects of their identity that they have already established.

The importance that we place on any of our identities is partly dependent upon the extent to which we receive both intrinsic and extrinsic rewards for assuming such an identity. If an identity typically supports positive interactions with other people and helps us to develop strong ties with others, then we tend to rank that identity as fairly high in our hierarchy (Burke and Stets 2009). People may merge roles with their person when playing that role helps them feel particularly good about themselves and those roles are positively evaluated. The more benefits associated with playing a particular role will increase the tendency for the person to experience a role merger (Turner 1978). For many participants, belly dance provides a wide range of rewards that I have discussed throughout this book, such as community, exercise, body acceptance, gender performance, recognition, and spirituality. Therefore, they are motivated to learn and abide by general community and group-specific norms. At the same time, there are costs that accompany identifying with some subcultures, and a variety of difficulties can threaten a belly dance identity. These challenges are the focus of the next two chapters.

Chapter 7

"There's enough drama in belly dance"

Browsing on Facebook one evening, Margot, a relatively new and young dancer sends me a message. An acquaintance of hers has asked her to perform at a private party. She wants to accept the invitation because she loves dancing and wants to support her friend, but she hesitates. "Will I step on any local dancers' toes?" she asks me. As she is not from the area in which the party is to take place, neither of us are familiar with the local dance scene in that community. As a dancer with only a few years of experience, she does not want to anger more advanced dancers and risk being ostracized. Some dancers want to maintain ownership over their dance "turf." In other words, some dancers are regular performers in particular venues or are considered the most sought-after performer should a performance opportunity in a particular geographic area arise. Dancers who do not want to risk offending other participants are careful to seek out opportunities that are not already considered part of another dancer's "turf." After considering her question for a few seconds, I respond that since she is not dancing in a public restaurant, the party is not an ongoing event in which she may be replacing a regular dancer, the gathering is a private event that probably few other people know about, and she is not actively soliciting dance employment, I don't see many turf issues with this situation. Reflecting on how other dancers may judge her if she were to accept this opportunity, Margot illustrates her desire not to steal a performance opportunity from another dancer. Learning and abiding by these informal rules related to status and legitimacy is an integral part of a dancer's socialization to maintain positive relationships with other dancers.

Much interactionist work touches on how people enact power relations and how conflicting parties compete and negotiate with one another (Dennis and Martin 2005). Power permeates all of our relationships and experiences (Foucault 1976). Power struggles, legitimacy claims, boundary work, and status hierarchies are some of the most difficult situations that affect belly dance communities. Some participants experience a host of passive aggressive behaviors from other members in the community, such as backstabbing, undercutting, gig-stealing, and cattiness. All of these negative behaviors violate norms within the world of belly dance.

Power dynamics and boundary work

Group members who wield greater amounts of power establish and enforce the rules for the entire collectivity. These varying "abilities to make rules and apply them to other people" are known as power differentials (Dennis and Martin 2005:199). The main structural positions of power within belly dance are class teacher, workshop instructor, and troupe leader (see Figure 7.1). Quite often some or all of these positions overlap. For instance, someone who teaches regular classes may also direct a troupe and occasionally teach workshops. The major power differences in belly dance occur between students and teachers and/or troupe leaders and troupe members. Boundaries are created around who may and may not legitimately occupy leadership roles, and norms dictate how teachers, troupe leaders, troupe members, and students should be treated.

Classroom instructors and troupe leaders wield power in several ways. Instructors occasionally offer multiple classes for students with different levels of dance experience and ability consisting of beginner, intermediate, and advanced. Based on their generally agreed upon skills and experiences, instructors are typically viewed by other dancers as having legitimate authority (Weber 1958). Teachers occasionally make decisions regarding when students may advance to the next level of classes. Instructors also decide when their students may perform and join performance troupes. Just as some students advance to higher level classes before others, some students are asked to join troupes before others. Students generally respect the judgment of their

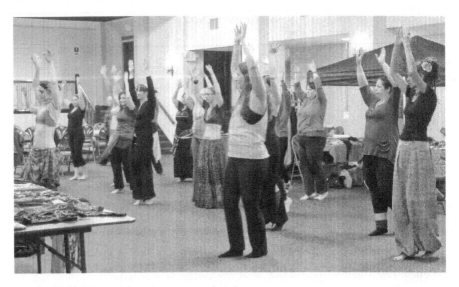

Figure 7.1 Workshop with an instructor and students

124

teachers and troupe leaders. Pointing out how various instructors have different goals for their groups, Dena states, "I let my students perform much earlier than some other instructors."

In some communities, boundaries are drawn between student troupes and their more advanced counterparts, or mother troupes (sometimes considered a professional troupe). Cynthia Fuchs Epstein (1992:233) defines boundaries as "the social territories of human relations, signaling who ought to be admitted and who excluded." Symbolic boundaries, such as words, ideas, or images draw lines between groups, and these groups typically have different access to power, resources, and status (Lamont and Molnar 2002; Swarts 2011). In some communities, the student troupe and mother troupe (also known as main, primary, or lead) are kept separate. Although members of each may perform separately, members of the different troupes may rarely perform together, the student troupe may not perform as often as the main troupe, and the student troupe may not be a "feeder" experience for membership in the mother troupe. In other cases, members of each troupe frequently dance together so there is little discernible difference between memberships in the different troupes. In these cases, belonging to a student troupe may also be a stepping stone to eventually joining the main troupe. Nonetheless, troupe leaders, sometimes in consultation with existing troupe members, decide who and when a dancer may join a student troupe and advance from a student troupe to the main troupe.

Similar to video game players (Khanolkar and McLean 2012), belly dancers are distinguished by status characteristics. A status characteristic is an attribute to which value and competence are attached, such as sex, age, or education (Correll and Ridgeway 2003). Status characteristics and different abilities contribute to inequalities within groups. Members with higher status and greater ability tend to receive more rewards than their counterparts (Melamed 2013). Fine (1987:95) uses the term "ability gradient" to refer to different abilities of members in a social group. Whether it is evaluating one's skill level to be part of a troupe, to perform, or to offer instruction, many belly dancers are judged and ranked based on their abilities. Dancers who are determined to have greater abilities receive higher rewards in the form of troupe membership, performance opportunities, and invitations to teach classes. About the professional troupe she leads, Ariel says, "It's far more indicative of the skill level, both technique and performance presence, that I expect from troupe members. The troupe shows off everyone's hard-earned skills that I consider to be of a professional caliber."

"I used to call her the nasty teacher"

Students learn belly dance movements, etiquette, culture, history, costuming, and choreography from teachers. Teachers are important sources of information, disseminators of knowledge, and technique instructors. Therefore, disrespecting teachers is looked down upon and violates an informal norm of deference to and respect of one's instructor. As a seasoned dancer and frequent workshop leader for over thirty-five years, Lana has had numerous interactions with students who have attempted to divert attention away from her to showcase their own knowledge or dance abilities. "There's always one idiot who comes and wants to show everybody that they know more than you do and show how smart they are and want to show off," Lana tells me. Lana reframes these situations as interactions she anticipates. "Come on in, come on in. I've been expecting you," Lana says quietly to herself during these confrontations. "How do you handle those students?" I inquire. "I start off really nice, and I say, 'wow that's a really good point! Thank you for bringing that up' or 'obviously you've given this a lot of thought' or 'it looks like you've done some homework, and you've read a lot on the subject.'" Responding in this way gives the dancer the attention she is most likely seeking and it allows Lana to avoid a power struggle. Occasionally, she ignores people who constantly interrupt her class. Although she does not tolerate students disrupting her instruction, Lana attempts to work with difficult situations because she believes a teacher has a great deal of responsibility toward her students.

Because instructors hold power, they are incredibly influential and can make or break a person's experience with belly dance. "The teacher generates the climate in the classroom. If she is threatened and competitive and angry then the students will be influenced by that," Lana says. "Teachers don't realize how much power they wield in a classroom. Even not intentionally you can cut a student by saying something thoughtless," Lana elaborates.

Cameron's experience with her first instructor illustrates the negative influence an instructor can have on her students. She describes her teacher as "extremely opinionated." "She doesn't use a filter in what she is thinking and what comes out of her mouth," Cameron tells me. Her former teacher offended numerous students. Cameron remembers her being "abrasive, rude, and inconsiderate." Rather than a democratic collectivity, the instructor managed her classes using a top-down approach and expected the students to do whatever she told them to do without incorporating any suggestions. It didn't take Cameron long to feel uncomfortable in that group. "About six months later I ended up leaving the troupe," Cameron says.

When Barbara had some strained interactions with her instructor, she also took a break from belly dance. She recalls feeling like classes with that teacher were repetitive and "like I wasn't learning anything new." It was so frustrating for her that "I just thought I was fed up with belly dance." However, Barbara realized that she was probably more unsatisfied with her teacher than with belly dance. Like Cameron, Barbara remembers her teacher being "mean." "I used to call her the nasty teacher," Barbara recalls. "What the hell do you think you are doing?" Barbara says, mimicking her screaming instructor. Although she was rarely the direct target of her teacher's wrath, Barbara's ego would take a hit any time her instructor would get upset. For a while, Barbara ceased her participation in belly dance because she did not like her teacher's instruction and she did not have a strong relationship with her teacher. Barbara has since found instructors with whom she "clicks" and continues her involvement in belly dance now as an instructor and troupe director. Both Barbara's and Cameron's experiences illustrate that a teacher's power is not unconditionally accepted by all students all of the time. In both cases, strained interactions with teachers caused Barbara and Cameron to re-evaluate their participation in belly dance.

"She started teaching when she was younger"

Students view instructors and troupe leaders as having a greater level of ability, experience, and expertise than them. It is generally understood that instructors and troupe leaders have been involved in dance for an extended length of time. Therefore, when people offer lessons or manage a troupe relatively early in their dance experience, they are viewed as violating a norm that a certain amount of time should elapse before anyone teaches belly dance. A dancer's legitimacy as an instructor is partly determined by her age, the amount of time she has been dancing, and the extent of her own training. Although some people offer dance instruction much earlier in their dance experience, there remain unspoken rules about when someone may legitimately become a belly dance instructor.

I have dinner one night with my department Chair and two reviewers as part of a department self-study. The conversation turns to my writing this book. My department Chair mentions my faculty advisor role of my university's belly dance club. "Do you teach lessons?" one reviewer inquires. Without hesitation, and probably with more force than the question requires, I quickly answer, "absolutely not." I explain that there are informal rules in the belly dance community about who should and should not teach. When the belly dance club was formed, there were more experienced dancers teaching in the area. Because I have never taught lessons, and I do not have comparable skills as the instructors in the area, I would not be judged as a legitimate teacher. Furthermore, I may be viewed as trying to steal students from more experienced and established teachers around my hometown. Rather than attempting to take business, the club has implemented several gatekeeping mechanisms to protect the local instructors.

Gatekeepers establish and enforce rules and norms. They draw boundaries around what is considered legitimate behavior and limit the voice of people

127

who do not adhere to those norms (Shaw 2012). Club members take lessons from resident teachers rather than from me or other group members. In fact, taking lessons from one of several local belly dance teachers is a requirement for club members to participate in some club activities and to perform in certain shows. This arrangement partially functions to support local dance teachers, which ideally minimizes feelings of competition between them and the club.

Before a performance, I see Hyacinth, a dancer friend of mine, in the women's restroom adjacent to the hall where we are both dancing that evening. I have not spoken to her in a while since she moved. "Were you taking belly dance classes?" I ask her from the common area while she finishes changing into her costume, applying makeup, and styling her hair. "Yes, I took classes with [an instructor], but there's a lot of controversy surrounding that dancer. Some people don't like her very much," she explains. I wonder why this is the case. "Well, she started teaching when she was [young]," Hyacinth replies. Her instructor began offering lessons at a younger age than many of the dancers in her area deem legitimate. In the belly dance community, age is one rough indicator of how much experience, and hence, status a dancer has. Instructors who are relatively "older," more experienced, and judged more talented than other dancers in the same general area are granted higher status and are seen as more legitimate teachers.

Although Laurel had only been involved in belly dance for less than a year, she was asked to teach dance classes. However, she sensed that some dancers in her area disapproved of the offer. If a dancer is invited to teach or perform without having the experience some others believe is necessary, those people may disapprove of the dancer accepting the invitation. Some dancers feel slighted if they are passed over for a teaching or performance opportunity that they think they should have. Unfortunately, "The claws came out," Laurel recalls. "I guess it was jealousy." There is a status hierarchy in which Laurel's teacher has been dancing for thirty years and is much older than Laurel; therefore, she holds more status than Laurel in her geographic area. As someone with more status, Laurel's teacher may feel entitled to greater rewards, such as being offered the additional teaching opportunity before Laurel. As a result, Laurel "chose not to go back there because it got downright nasty." She did not accept the teaching offer even though "I would have loved to have done it. This is like a dream come true for me." However, Laurel remembers that only a few other dancers in her area would speak to her because of their allegiance to her now former teacher. "I just didn't want to have that about my name," she explains.

"She's just not happy with herself, so she just likes to lash out at other people. She likes to write things on her website about how the other teachers in [the area] are not qualified, and they don't know what they are doing," Julia tells me about an instructor in her town. "What kinds of things does she write on her website?" I inquire. "Be careful when you are picking out a teacher because some of them are not qualified and you could hurt yourself because they just don't know how to teach," Julia explains. Although these warnings about choosing qualified instructors may be fair and reasonable, who is and who isn't qualified to teach belly dance is mostly subjective. By making comments about who she thinks is and isn't qualified to teach, the instructor to whom Julia refers attempts to draw boundaries around legitimate and illegitimate teachers. With the exception of an established American Tribal Style curriculum and its official training program, there are no set credentials that dancers have to earn before they can offer belly dance instruction. Rather there is an informal legitimacy code. All of these examples point to norms about who should and should not be teaching.

"I'm not invited to go to something because of other people I dance with"

Partly due to loyalty to one's dance teacher, some dancers do not seek out other instructors even if those teachers radically alter the style of dance they teach. Norma has danced with her instructor for about two years when we talk. Her teacher began offering lessons in a new dance style. Rather than seeking a different teacher and continue taking lessons in the style to which she was accustomed, Norma elected to remain with her teacher and learn a new form of dance. Although some instructors encourage their students to take classes from many different teachers, "It would have been awkward if I was in another troupe," Norma replies to my inquiry about remaining with her instructor. "Just some problems that have been experienced. Some different fractions would make it awkward to be in this troupe and take classes from someone else," Norma continues. If Norma were to leave her group and start taking lessons with another teacher who has a strained relationship with her current instructor, Norma could be guilty by association, which could cause difficulties between her and her teacher.

The potential conflict that Norma surmises is not completely imagined. "I've had someone tell me that I'm not invited to go to something because of other people I dance with," Julia explains. Similar to establishing boundaries, Julia's experiences are indicative of "borderwork," which refers to conceptual distinctions made between parties (Thorne 1993). It is not uncommon for belly dance troupes to cross geographic boundaries to participate in events with other troupes. However, they are occasionally met with resistance thereby reinforcing boundaries between troupes. Affiliation with different groups becomes a basis for categorizing people (Lamont and Molnar 2002) and membership in a particular group becomes a reason to exclude someone from an event. Sponsoring groups control access to those events and have the power to decide who may perform and who is excluded.

Despite multiple groups in an area, "You go on to a tribe's website and they say they are the only official troupe in [the city]. Typically when you define a group that way, it's against a relevant out group," Scarlett astutely observes, which is not surprising given that she has advanced degrees in the social sciences. Scarlett keenly points out that by a group defining themselves as the only official troupe in an area, they create boundaries between themselves and other groups. They make legitimacy claims by suggesting that the other groups are not "real" belly dancers. Establishing boundaries leads to reflecting on negative aspects of an out-group, while valuing one's in-group (Bourdieu 1984; Lamont 1992; Taylor 2002). Norma, Julia, and Scarlett's experiences all illustrate how boundaries are drawn between in-groups and out-groups.

"She should be kissing my ass"

Informal norms regarding who or what troupe has more rank are partly determined by who has been in an area the longest and the rights and privileges that accompany being an established dancer. "Are there any challenges you experience in belly dance that are bigger issues now that when you first started?" I ask Meredith. "You have to play the politics," Meredith replies. After being involved in belly dance for over five years, Meredith says, "You have to kiss ass, and you have to make sure you don't offend other dancers, especially the ones who've been around longer. I'm anti-politics, and it's been a real challenge for me." I ask her for an example. "Making sure you invite the right people to the right events, and if they invite you just saying 'Oh thank you very much,'" Meredith replies. Meredith tells me about a show at which she performed that took place on the top floor of a building that had no air conditioning "with sweat dripping down my legs." Because Meredith was terribly uncomfortable the entire evening, she felt disrespected that the event coordinator didn't show more concern for the performers. "I am still furious about it. I've been in the community longer than she has, and she should be kissing my ass, but she is clueless. She is kind of a baby belly dancer, and I feel like she got too much power too fast." Meredith's comments illustrate her belief that length of time in the belly dance community grants her some amount of seniority and respect from other dancers. A "baby belly dancer" is someone who is relatively new to belly dance and has been dancing for less than five to seven years, although this amount of time is fluid. Along with being sure to invite the "right" people, groups navigate the scheduling of their events with some concern for "first come first serve" and the "seniority" of groups.

It is not uncommon for multiple belly dance groups to exist in the same city, even small cities. Groups generally take care not to schedule events that overlap with programs in surrounding areas because belly dance events typically draw from similar crowds. If too many events occur simultaneously, audiences may spread out and attendance at any one event may be lower. Having low attendance at events can be problematic for groups because they may not have enough paying attendees to recover the costs associated with hosting an event (room rents, equipment rental, hired assistance, etc.). Furthermore, some groups host fundraisers to help fellow dancers with medical bills and/or challenging familial situations (as described in Chapter 4). Having fewer people in attendance means less money raised to help those in need.

Amber and I discuss some problems that arose when her group advertised a performance on the same day that another troupe in her area hosted an event. "Was this competition between the groups?" I ask. The other group is "more established," according to Amber. "They have been around longer . . . and we had something big going on and then these other people ended up having a benefit for this belly dancer who has breast cancer. I am like, 'Oh my gosh, are you really going to bring charity into this little squabble?' Of course [attendees] are going to go to a hafla that is supporting this dancer with breast cancer instead of coming to our thing, which we planned first." Although Amber's group organized an event first, the other troupe was more established and hosted an event that some may view as more meaningful compared to Amber's group's event. As Amber illustrates, tension can sometimes arise when different groups want to host events in the same area. Informal norms dictate that when planning an event, the organizer tries to avoid setting a date that competes with other belly dance events in close geographical proximity.

The battle for paid performances

Performance opportunities are limited, and paid performances are scarcer still. There are only so many restaurants or events at which belly dancers perform, especially in smaller towns. Because many dancers enjoy performing and there are scant numbers of performance outlets, not having those opportunities can lead to an undercurrent of hostility and hurt feelings between some dancers. Those dancers holding more power can exert some control over who performs (sometimes for pay) and who doesn't.

I sit quietly as Avery fills out a brief survey. While reading the questionnaire, she begins to snicker, so I look at the paper to see what question she is answering and make a mental note to inquire about that question during our chat. After Avery finishes the survey and we begin our talk, I ask her, "Why did you chuckle at the question about being an amateur?" "Last week, I danced at a restaurant," Avery begins. The owner of the establishment told Avery that a woman in the audience wanted to perform. "I talked with her and maybe she is a beginner . . . She has taken like two classes, and she considers herself a belly dancer enough to dance at the restaurant. I mean she did have some moves, but they weren't clear. I don't think I would have danced at a restaurant after two classes." Similar to expectations regarding teaching, Avery's reaction illustrates unspoken norms about when it is appropriate to perform in restaurants.

Avery schedules the dancers at this Middle Eastern restaurant. When making decisions about who performs, Avery tries to give her friends and people she knows priority for dancing opportunities. "I still will do as the restaurant requests if they [greatly enjoy someone's dancing]." If the restaurant is less enthusiastic about a dancer, she will get placed on an "alternate" list and will only be called if a regularly scheduled dancer is not able to perform on a given night. Avery shares some degree of control with the restaurant owners over who and when dancers perform at the restaurant. But, decisions made by both the restaurant owners and Avery require judgment about different dancers' abilities, and this is not always comfortable for Avery. "There is a bit of guilt associated with having to rank dancers and worry about their feelings if the restaurant asks that they not dance or that they be on the alternate list. I know I hate judging other dancers for the restaurant," Avery continues. Although there is only one dancer per evening at the restaurant, "sometimes there is awkwardness if one dancer is given more nights than another or one is given Fridays versus Saturdays," Avery tells me. "Are Fridays or Saturdays viewed as more prestigious or meant for the top dancers?" I ask. Although Avery does not think there is much difference between the two days, some dancers believe that Saturdays are busier and present more opportunities to earn tips. Not only does Avery make decisions about who will dance at a restaurant, she also has to navigate dancers' perceptions regarding prime dance times and make decisions about who to schedule on what evenings.

"They were undercutting people's prices so badly"

Few friendships form in tango clubs because many dancers prioritize their own self-interest. Because they do not feel committed to other dancers, there is little trust between dancers and they often question each other's motives (Savigliano 1998). People wonder if dancers are stealing new steps for a show or attempting to get hired for an event (Savigliano 1998). Although the setting is a little different in that much of American belly dance exists in semi-private classes, troupes, and events rather than public clubs, some dancers are cautious of other dancers stealing income opportunities, such as paid performances and/or paying students.

The lack of paid performance opportunities partly inflames competition and conflict between dancers. Belly dance is not cheap. As I described in Chapter 1, dancers spend money on classes, workshops, videos, costumes, makeup, hair accessories, and props. Despite the potentially large financial investment in the activity, few dancers make a living at belly dance. It is challenging, if not impossible, to recover much of the money one invests in the dance. Any opportunity that a dancer has to earn at least some money is highly coveted. It is expected that dancers in the same area will charge comparable prices for their performances and teaching. Unfortunately, not all dancers adhere to these norms.

Undercutting occurs when a dancer or a group accepts substantially lower pay for a performance than the standard rate in a particular area. Some may offer to dance for free and/or for tips collected during their show. "It got to the point that they were undercutting people's prices so badly that [restaurant and other venue owners] would start calling us back up and say 'Oh I found this other group to do it,'" Grace tells me about her experience with one group. "It was bad because one of the things we try to do is hold a price standard among all of us. Everyone tries to charge the same thing." Because of norms dictating that comparable prices are charged for similar services, when a group accepts a lower amount of money for a performance than the local rate, "that really left a bad taste in all our mouths," says Grace. Furthermore, this group also attends performances of other dancers and distributes their own business cards for future events attempting to replace the group that was already performing in that establishment.

Sydney tells me about a dancer who will not perform in the same venue where she dances. "What do you think the issue is that this dancer has with you?" I ask Sydney. "There is your beginning belly dance, your middle, and then there is that age where it is really beautiful to look at those women, in their forties and fifties, if she is comfortable with her body and moving it," Sydney replies. She suggests that this dancer is aging and "trying so hard to compete with [Sydney] instead of being comfortable in her body and portraying where she is in this stage of her life," Sydney surmises. Sydney suggests that this dancer is competitive with younger dancers, and may not want to dance where Sydney dances because Sydney is younger than she is. Sydney is also stereotypically attractive. She is tall and thin with long blonde hair and a captivating smile, which may also intimidate an older dancer. Sydney's comments mirror the experiences of some "table-dancers" for whom aging diminishes their desirability and ability to earn money (Ronai 1992). One strategy that some "table-dancers" use to protect their involvement in the business and earning potential is to move to other bars where they are younger and more attractive compared to other dancers (Ronai 1992). The dancer to whom Sydney refers may use a similar strategy by no longer dancing in the same location as Sydney.

Interestingly, I did not talk to a single male who experiences any competition or undercutting for gigs. During our chat, Henry tells me that he isn't treated differently as a male belly dancer, but he feels unique in terms of access to public performance opportunities (as opposed to an event with primarily a belly dance audience). A Turkish restaurant in Henry's town hires belly dancers to perform. However, Henry believes "they will never hire me" because the owner is a "traditional Turkish guy." "Traditional Turkish men do not want to see a male belly dancer," Henry explains. "So my choice of gigs is a little limited." On the other hand, Henry recognizes that having a different set of performance opportunities means he has a different interaction dynamic with other dancers compared to his female counterparts. "There's a bit of cattiness and competiveness among the women who are competing for gigs," Henry begins. "I'm never going to be competing for the exact same gigs as my female friends." Not having to compete with other dancers over paid performance opportunities means that Henry does not experience the gig-stealing and undercutting that many female performers do. In some ways, he and other male dancers are protected from these competitive interactions and his friendships with female dancers are typically not threatened if he is chosen for a gig over them.

Catfighting

Girls' and women's groups can encourage nurturing and friendship (Green 1998), and many women receive support from their female colleagues (Jones and Palmer 2011). At the same time, research has documented ridicule and social exclusion within girls' play groups (Goodwin 2002) and animosity and competition among women at work (Dellasegra 2005; Jones and Palmer 2011; Mooney 2005; Tanenbaum 2002). Some women attempt to sabotage their female co-workers, spread rumors, gossip, experience jealousy, withhold friendships, and insult each other (Bearman *et al.* 2009; Crick *et al.* 2002; Mooney 2005; Tanenbaum 2002; Xie *et al.* 2002). These behaviors are known as "catfights," a "derogatory way to describe a vicious clash between women" (Tanenbaum, 2002:29).

Catfighting involves indirect aggression, which is more common in friendships than other kinds of more permanent relationships, such as families (Tanenbaum 2002). Direct, more than indirect, aggression is likely to damage interactions. Indirect aggressive techniques are used to try to preserve some aspect of the connection (Brown 2003; Richardson 2005). Furthermore, because people tend to compare themselves to other members of their groups, they are more likely to compete with people who are only slightly more advantaged than themselves and warrant social comparison. For instance, women tend to compete more with other women, rather than with men, partly because they do not see men as true rivals (Bearman *et al.* 2009; Tanenbaum 2002). Often women do not feel they strive for the same things as men or they recognize that men generally have more power and privilege than women (Tanenbaum 2002). In belly dance, this lack of competition between men and women is evident in Henry's comments.

Some belly dancers make and/or have received derogatory comments about another dancer's appearance or ability. Statements about how a dancer looks can be a form of "internalized sexism," which occurs when women behave toward other women in sexist ways they have learned from society. As I discussed in Chapter 3, due to the plethora of media that showcase the female body, women are regularly evaluated on how they look and quickly learn the value placed on appearance. When women internalize sexism, they judge their own and each other's appearance as they become both observer and evaluator (Bearman *et al.* 2009).

A dancer friend of Lana's is a "very nice dancer, with magnificent red hair," Lana fondly recalls. Since this dancer's hair almost touched the floor, Lana deems it a "show stopper." During the performances at the amusement park at which Lana and her friend danced, each dancer would perform a solo act. Some of the dancers "were mean and would claim that when she was spinning, her hair would hit people, so they would duck in this exaggerated way," Lana remembers. These dancers asked the group leader to force the dancer to pin her hair up. In this way, these girls were acting like "fashion police" (Simmons 2011) by attempting to control this dancer's appearance and condemning her when they thought she did not conform to their expectations. They were also ganging up on her, a fairly common strategy that girls use to display indirect aggression toward other girls (Simmons 2011). But, "it wasn't hitting anybody," Lana explains. Rather, the dancers who complained "didn't want [Lana's friend] getting all this attention because her hair was just magnificent," according to Lana.

Similar to Lana's friend, some dancers made insulting comments about a costume Grace wore at a belly dance association's gathering many years ago. "I don't know if they were jealous or what, but [other dancers attending the event] were so mean to me when I first started," Grace recalls. In fact, "I quit [the organization] . . . I didn't want to dance with [the group] anymore." "What could have happened that would push you to leave the organization?" I ask. "I was way ahead of my time in fashion, and one of the girls came around and was gawking at me," Grace remembers. One dancer snidely said to her, "You're not going to wear that on stage are you?" "I was crushed," Grace remembers. However, she was determined to go out on stage and "knock 'em dead." Although she performed to her satisfaction, "I decided I was going to distance myself from those kinds of people," Grace tells me. Similar to Cameron and

Barbara who took temporary breaks from belly dance when they had difficulty getting along with their teachers, Grace quit her dance association "and for a long time, it was hard for me to be a part of the community of dancers." Also like Barbara and Cameron, Grace eventually found a friendlier group of dancers and continues her involvement in belly dance today.

Although the people that Grace encountered may not have been reprimanded for their behavior, some other dancers report feeling the need to censor derogatory comments. With the exception of power differentials between teacher and student, an informal rule within belly dance is that all dancers are relatively equal in status, although experience and ability (real or perceived) may distinguish some dancers from others. Maggie attempts to control feelings of superiority that occasionally arise among her dance students. "I think there's a possibility for the diva attitude to really flourish in belly dancing because when you get onstage you have to have the diva attitude," Maggie tells me. A belly dance diva is overly confident and, at times, believes she is a better dancer or performer than her peers. Maggie believes that, to some degree, dancers must have that confidence in order to be able to dance on stage, especially if they perform solos. However, she stresses that the confidence and feeling like "I'm awesome" needs to be "saved specifically for the stage. It should not come off the stage ever!" Maggie exclaims. A few members of Maggie's group started to develop diva personalities outside of performing and "we just nip it in the bud. We don't allow it," Maggie says. Like other dance instructors and troupe leaders, Maggie has the authority to enforce expectations of relative equality among her dancers. Reprimanding students is one example of how some dancers manage catty behavior.

Authentic belly dance

Some of the tension that arises between dancers stems from debates regarding who is a legitimate belly dancer and whether one's participation is "authentic." "Authenticity ... refers to a set of qualities that people in a particular time and place have come to agree represent an ideal or exemplar" (Vannini and Williams 2009:3). As such, authenticity can be a marker of status (Vannini and Williams 2009). Authenticity of participants' behaviors and identities is hotly contested in a number of subcultures, such as straightedge (Williams 2006), hip-hop and rap (Harkness 2012; Harrison 2008), Goth and wannabes (Wilkins 2008), and the skateboard scene (Dupont 2014). Some members of the Pagan community wrestle with issues of authenticity as they draw from a variety of cultural and ethnic resources to establish their identities (Magliocco 2004). For instance, some Pagans attempt to reclaim pre-Christian traditions from Europe and borrow traditions from other cultures, such as Native Americans. They also attempt to establish authenticity through ties to various cultural traditions and develop personal relationships with people belonging to the cultures from which they borrow. Rooted in these beliefs is the idea that some cultures are the territory of certain people. However, Magliocco (2004) argues that although we usually think about racial and ethnic categories as having definitive properties, they are fluid. Rather than being set in stone, these categories morph, change, and are reinvented over time. Furthermore, cultural heritage can be considered a form of art, and art forms are susceptible to cross-cultural influences, blending, and reshaping (Magliocco 2004). Much like some Pagans, belly dancers occasionally debate the authenticity of their participation in this world.

Discussions of authenticity can only happen within a context of set conventions. Like ballroom (Marion 2008), some participants have firm ideas about what constitutes belly dance. Accepted norms provide guidelines and standards for music, movement, and costume. Dancers may want to "push the envelope" to stand out and express themselves, but doing so too much may raise questions about the legitimacy of one's belly dance. Performances that stray too far from accepted dance may invite accusations from other dancers that these creative acts violate norms surrounding appropriate music and dance.

Participation in a community may be judged problematic if one is deemed inauthentic (Nowotny et al. 2010). Some forms of Latin music are viewed as less authentic compared to other types partly due to the participation of Anglos (Nowotny et al. 2010). Likewise, although its roots are in Middle Eastern culture and ways of life in surrounding areas, belly dance in the United States is an activity dominated by "white" women, which has caused serious controversy in the community across the country.

On March 6, 2014, Randa Jarrar published an online article titled "Why I Can't Stand White Belly Dancers." Jarrar discusses her life growing up in the Middle East and the role of Raqs Sharqi, as belly dance is known in its areas of origin. She shares her discomfort with white women in "Arab drag" as she calls some restaurant performers in the United States. She objects to the costumes, makeup, and stage names that some dancers adopt and refers to white women using these props as "browning" and appropriating Middle Eastern dance. There was a flood of responses across many Internet sites defending the participation of white women in belly dance. Putting aside the issue of cultural appropriation, I am more concerned with the underlining assumptions regarding authenticity, claims about who should and should not belly dance, and the potential violation of community norms.

Authenticity is socially constructed (Vannini and Williams 2009). As illustrated in Jarrar's article, some dancers judge various styles of belly dance as more authentic than others. One characteristic that influences whether music and dance are deemed authentic is the degree to which they are steeped in tradition. Conjunto is Latin music closely tied to tradition, and fans enjoy it partly because it helps them connect to and share their past. Conversely, salsa and jazz are newer types of Latin music, and are deemed less authentic (Nowotny *et al.* 2010). Likewise, the American Tribal Style and tribal fusion styles of belly dance are relatively recent creations and deemed less authentic compared to traditional Middle Eastern dances that some claim are thousands of years old. As one American Tribal Style dancer observes, "we are very welcoming of [Middle Eastern style dancers], but they are more likely to snub us."

Along with being rooted in tradition, authenticity of dance is partly tied to the extent to which it is formal and codified. The two less authentic forms of Latin music are also more formalized, while traditional Latin music involves spontaneous dancing (Nowotny *et al.* 2010). Likewise, the American Tribal Style has a codified set of movements and instructors become certified to teach this dance style. The American Tribal Style is based on improvisational dance in that routines are not tightly choreographed. American Tribal Style dancers learn cues, movements, and rules about when to perform particular steps. Traditional Middle Eastern belly dance has fewer rules, is not focused around a set curriculum of movements, and is often a solo and spontaneous dance.

Nearing the end of our two-hour conversation, I ask Dena, "Is there anything that could take you away from belly dance?" She replies, "If anything has made me want to quit, it would be where tribal fusion is going." Dena believes that "the biggest threat to belly dance today is the inability of people in the tribal fusion area to gauge themselves in any way to keep a connection with [traditional Middle Eastern dance]." She thinks some fusion dancers believe "I can do anything I darn well please and call it belly dance." "What is belly dance to you?" I ask Dena. With the confidence of a dancer and instructor of over thirty years, she replies:

> Belly dance is intrinsically tied to the Middle Eastern and North African cultures, and you can't have true belly dance without an awareness and a respectful treatment of the musical and terpsichorean aspects of those cultures. So, no, I do not view tribal, tribal fusion, gothic, steampunk, burlesque/belly combinations, etc. as belly dance. When you remove [Middle East and North Africa] aspects that govern those dances – the rhythms and musical compositions especially, but also the cultural connections – you take the dance outside belly dance.

Dena uses a few different strategies to implement her preferences for Middle Eastern and North African dance. With her students, "I do make my feelings known about what I believe is true belly dance and what is not, and why I believe it is so, from the very beginning." Dena tells students to practice to whatever music they wish, but "now I add, *just* [her emphasis] for practice, not for performance," she tells me. Furthermore, when Dena hosts an event showcasing several dancers, she tries to limit the number of non-Middle Eastern dance numbers and doesn't allow any alternative pieces in a folkloric show. In addition, Dena tells dancers from outside of her immediate group who are interested in performing at her events "that I am a purist and don't really like non-Middle Eastern music, so if someone wants to use such, they need to get it approved by me first." With both her students and guest dancers, Dena creates boundaries around the music that she deems appropriate for her shows. Likewise she acts as a gatekeeper to minimize her audience's exposure to non-Middle Eastern music and styles of belly dance.

"Is Middle Eastern dance an art form in your opinion?" I ask Dena. "I think it can be, but that's not what it is to me. To me it's passion," she responds. Dena believes that when something is defined as art, "the door opens for that creative license." For Dena, calling belly dance an art form loosens the boundaries of the dance and renders it subject to creative interpretation. But, when Dena labels Middle Eastern dance as culture and tradition, it is less subject to creativity. In these ways, Dena and others engage in a reality definition contest (Loseke 1987) regarding what is and isn't belly dance. Dena's definitions of belly dance prevail in situations where she maintains power and control over the setting, such as in her classroom or events that she sponsors. Similar to dancers like Dena and Jarrar, some Pagans are concerned about cultural appropriation in their communities. Some members of the community are perceived to be not as sensitive to and respectful of the original cultures and traditions from which they borrow (Magliocco 2004).

For reasons similar to Dena's concerns regarding cultural appropriation, Scarlett eventually left belly dance. After a few years of taking classes, Scarlett removed herself from the community when she reconceptualized belly dance and her new perspective clashed with her values. Since leaving the activity, Scarlett comments, "A lot of it might be this illusion with the cultural appropriation that I feel goes on with belly dance." "What do you mean by cultural appropriation?" I inquire. Scarlett refers to the controversies surrounding sports teams using Native American names and mascots. "They feel like they are honoring the culture by having this white person dress up as an Indian and dance like one for their sports team, and it's not. It's not even honoring a culture because it's not really their culture. It's what these white people think is their culture," Scarlett explains. Scarlett likens belly dance in America to "a concurring nation." In other words, she believes people from Middle Eastern and North African countries "probably wouldn't appreciate us pretending that we're one of them."

However, some American Tribal Style and tribal fusion dancers interpret concerns for authenticity as judgments that divide dancers. Alicia says, "Some people are like, if you're not doing, for example, Egyptian, you're not doing true belly dance. I don't believe that. It's all fun. It's all good. It's an evolving art form . . . There can be some conflict with different people who aren't supportive of the different styles." For dancers like Alicia, belly dance is an art form, and, as Dena suggested, labeling belly dance as an art form allows for creativity and interpretation.

"Is belly dance an art, culture, tradition, or something else?" I ask Mona, an American Tribal Style dancer. "For me, belly dance is another form of dance, which has roots in culture and tradition, but is also an art form," Mona replies. "Painting and sculpture were once rooted in culture and tradition, some of it still is, but it has since blossomed into more than that. It has been picked up by those outside of the original cultures, who don't always know or even care about the traditions, who are looking at it in a new way. I think the same is true of dance." Illustrating Dena's concerns, some dancers focus less on cultural tradition and more on art.

Relationship challenges

Interpersonal strains within belly dance can be so challenging that some people exit the world of belly dance. Finding communities to which one feels connected is a core prerequisite for staying involved in belly dance. If a person no longer feels tied to a group, she or he may decide to leave belly dance. Describing some lessons she tried in her new city after a cross-country move, Emma says, "I went to a couple of classes there, but it was just stupid." Emma had some difficulty understanding the steps in the intermediate class she joined and "they were not welcoming at all." "I went twice to that class, and I don't know if they were cliquey or what. There also wasn't much conversation between sets or anything. I also got there before class to try and meet people, but no one was talking to anybody. So it was just kind of like this cold thing," Emma continues. The students in a different class were more pleasant, "but I knew more about tribal than they did. That's disturbing. I mean, they were nice and everything, but I wasn't going to get anything out of it." Emma tried yet another set of classes, but experiences there reminded her of some previous strained interactions with a few dancers in her prior city. As of the last time we chatted, Emma could not find a new belly dance group in which she felt comfortable and has ceased her participation in belly dance.

Belly dancers manage power struggles, questions of legitimacy, and status hierarchies. Boundaries are drawn between legitimate and illegitimate teachers, student and professional dancers, and authentic belly dance. Norms surround these boundaries, and violating them can cause friction. Judgments regarding dance ability separate amateur dancers from those talented enough to perform for pay. In-groups and out-groups, much like cliques, are established.

Although many of the challenges discussed in this chapter refer to interpersonal interactions, they are, to varying degrees, tied to the reality that belly dance is shared with the public. Belly dance is not hidden. Many instructors feel obligated to deliver a public performance that is as professional and polished as possible. These group leaders may limit performance opportunities to dancers they believe have the greatest ability and stage presence. Similar judgments are made regarding who performs at restaurants. Factors such as which dancers may attract patrons and provide entertainment that customers will enjoy are taken into account. Because the performance is shared with the general public, the focus ceases to be solely on the dancer's experience. Rather, instructors' concerns are whether an audience gets their money's worth of enjoyable entertainment. But how members of the general public perceive belly dancers is highly varied. In the next chapter, I investigate various consequences of the public nature of belly dance, particularly how both male and female participants manage some public perceptions of belly dancers.

Chapter 8

Negotiating erotic images of belly dance

When I begin taking belly dance classes in the fall of 2002, I hide my participation from the people in my academic department. As a graduate instructor, I am not much older than most of my students, and I am concerned about maintaining a professional image. My dance classes occur at a recreation center close to my university, and my group performs in the same area. I wonder if some of my students will perceive me differently if they attend a show and see me dance. Will I have difficulty managing my classroom as a result? I do not want to jeopardize my professional relationship with my students. Also, I am unsure how colleagues would view my participation in belly dance. I do not disclose my involvement to my dissertation committee, including my advisor. While I interview for academic positions during my last year of graduate school, I also hesitate to discuss my participation. Sharing my involvement in belly dance during one interview illustrates many dancers' concerns of being outed.

While visiting campuses, I give a research presentation based on my dissertation that examines the political priorities of religious lobbies on Capitol Hill (a far cry from belly dance). Immediately following the conclusion of my talk at one university, an audience member comments about the way I move around the room. In front of everyone, this person asks if I have a dance background. Apparently, I was caught a little offguard because this audience member also comments about my face turning bright red. Up until that point in my interview no one at the university knew about my involvement in belly dance. I silently reason that my participation in belly dance is eventually going to be known, especially since my future research agenda revolves heavily around the activity, so I announce that I take belly dance classes.

In hindsight, my apprehension about telling students, colleagues, and potential co-workers that I belly dance was probably unfounded. I never experienced any repercussions of which I am aware due to my involvement in the dance. But, these concerns are not uncommon. What is behind my behavior and the actions of many other participants is a general undercurrent of uneasiness that some members of the public liken belly dance to erotic dance, which is stigmatized in the United States. Regardless of how real the concerns may be, I and many other dancers act based on our assumptions and perceptions of how others may evaluate us.

Eroticizing belly dance

Although many participants use belly dance to do gender and express sensuality, some dancers simultaneously manage perceptions that belly dance is erotic dance. Like the internal power struggles that involve boundary work that I discussed in the previous chapter, dancers also engage in symbolic boundary work when negotiating external perceptions of belly dance. Members of religious fraternities are aware of negative connotations that accompany being part of the Greek system. They stereotype other fraternities as self-serving and focused on partying, which is different than the kinds of activities in which they participate (Gurrentz 2014). Also, rather than being viewed as sexualized beings, swimmers attempt to present an image that suggests they pursue fitness (Scott 2010). Like members of some fraternities and swimmers, belly dancers take the view of the other, evaluate themselves the way they think others may judge them, and attempt to present themselves in ways to manage how onlookers perceive them.

Cheryl tells me about a hafla she attended with her husband. During the show, her husband made one comment that illustrates the connection some members of the general public create between belly dance and erotic dance and the discomfort this association causes some dancers. Cheryl's husband remarked that belly dance "allows the inner stripper to come out of women legitimately. You know, it gives them that fulfillment," Cheryl recalls. Cheryl clearly did not appreciate her husband's insinuation as she exclaimed, "What do you mean inner stripper? Nobody is taking their clothes off," she retorted back. Similarly, many belly dancers define their performances as artistic and/or cultural entertainment, while some onlookers may construct the performance as erotic. Emphasizing not removing their clothes is one role-distance strategy, among many techniques, that belly dancers use to counteract perceptions that belly dance is like erotic dance.

"Talk about how belly dancers are similar to pole dancers," a colleague requests during one academic talk I give about belly dance. I am caught a little offguard, and I don't know how to respond to this inquiry. I do not conduct research on pole dancers, and I am not familiar with scholarly literature on pole dancing. Therefore, I am unclear about how belly dancers may or may not be similar to pole dancers. However, I am somewhat accustomed to separating belly dance from erotic dancers so, right or wrong, I interpret the question through that lens and attempt to symbolically separate belly dancers from my very limited, and probably somewhat naïve, impression of pole dancers. Distancing belly dance from erotic dance is a somewhat common strategy that some dancers use when interacting with the general public. The degree to which and how dancers work toward this separation varies by setting.

Context matters

Belly dancers perform in a variety of public places, such as on stages, in restaurants, libraries, hospitals, nursing homes, at festivals, and as part of cultural events (see Figures 8.1 and 8.2). To what extent and how participants play with the sexuality or sensuality of the dance hinge on both context and audience. Some dancers may construct their dance to be a little risqué in party contexts, such as some renaissance festivals, by flirting with audiences. Although these audiences are usually mixed, among them are people (particularly men) who have been drinking various intoxicating beverages and are part of a context that, in general, celebrates raunchiness.

There may be other venues (perhaps within the same event) in which dancers perform on a stage relatively separated from an audience and interactions may be more formal and less crude. In this sense, performing on a stage creates a particular set of interaction rules, while dancing among crowds suggests different norms. The informal guidelines that shape interactions within different settings create what is known as an "interaction membrane" (Goffman 1961). The interacting parties within a particular context create the rules for the encounter. To some degree, this may require the parties to reach a "working consensus" in that one party may not be fully on board with the rules emerging from the interaction, but rather than changing or leaving the interaction, the party decides to "play along" (Goffman 1959).

For example, throughout my over thirteen years of belly dance experience, there was only one instance where I felt objectified within a dance context. One evening, I, along with a few other dancers, performed at an outdoor event. Many of the attendees laugh and talk throughout our dancing. While performing in a set with three other dancers, some audience members not so quietly discuss, "Which one is your favorite?" We are sized up and compared to one another. During another set in which I dance a duet with one of my troupe

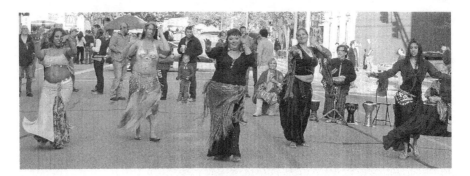

Figure 8.1 Dancers at a street festival

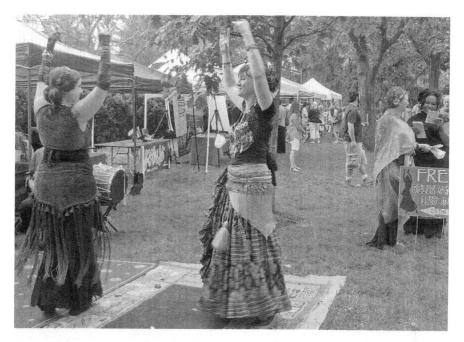

Figure 8.2 Dancers at an art festival

mates, we turn to face each other. We perform a body wave during which our right arm extends straight above our head, while our left is held in front of our chest and bent inward. We lean forward toward each other for the beginning of the body wave as I hear someone yell in the audience, "Kiss!" We lean our chests back completing the movement. I don't know how the other dancer feels, but I become very uncomfortable. However, I don't stop performing, and I never lecture the audience member about the inappropriateness of that comment. Rather, I play along with what appears to be the rules governing this particular context. This event impressed upon me the importance of context for establishing interaction rules and shaping management strategies.

A few days later, as I reflected on this event and discussed it with a few dancers, I realized there were several key components of the situation that were ripe for me feeling objectified. First, the event was at night, and the vast majority of the audience was men who had engaged in hypermasculine activities earlier in the day that reinforce traditional male characteristics of power and aggression. Second, the audience members were not familiar with belly dance, so they may have uninformed notions about what a belly dancer is. Third, many of the attendees were drinking, so much so that various containers of liquor and wine were passed around while people took turns drinking out of the bottles during our performances. Fourth, we danced in a very intimate setting under a tent (it was raining heavily) with the crowd sitting on blankets on the ground. We were so physically close to our audience that we contained our movements so as to not step on or run into anyone. Finally, in between our acts, we interacted with the audience, dancing, chatting, and laughing, and occasionally joining them for a drink. We were not just entertainers, we were part of the gathering. All of these factors coming together encouraged some audience members to behave in fairly raunchy ways toward us dancers.

Throughout her several decades of involvement in the dance, Marie has created numerous strategies to establish guidelines of interaction in the settings that may support objectification like this event. "I always make my dancers who think they'd like to do shimmy grams work with me to have a specific set of rules they relay to the hiring party, a set of questions they ask of the hiring party, and I insist that they never go alone!" Marie explains. Having these strategies, "helps cut down on the times someone decides you are fair game." But in contexts, such as the outdoor event, where we did not anticipate what the interactions would look like, "there's not much you can do . . . other than ignore, and walk away," the seasoned instructor tells me. Rather than walking away, I played along to some degree, with the interaction rules that became evident that evening. However, when we were not dancing our sets, I hung out in the back corner of the tent with some other dancers and the drummers who accompanied us away from the center of the interaction. This was my attempt to separate myself or "walk away" as much as I could without completely exiting the event.

Regardless of the strategies we employ, we cannot completely control eroticism. Erotic gazes happen every day in a heteronormative society in which heterosexual men gaze upon women regardless of the woman's intention of attracting that male gaze. Belly dance is saturated with intention. Few (if any) belly dancers perform in public with the intention of being erotic. Yet, regardless of a dancer's intention, some audiences may perceive her movements and/ or costume as erotic. As much as a dancer might wish to curtail the association between belly dance and erotic dance, her efforts may have limited influence on how some audiences perceive her. Nevertheless, as Marie demonstrates, dancers adopt various strategies to minimize the likelihood of being perceived as erotic.

Confronting stigma

Stigma occurs when a person possesses an attribute that is labeled different, and the difference is linked to a socially undesirable characteristic or negative stereotype (Goffman 1963; Link and Phelan 2001). As primarily a form of leisure, belly dance is voluntary and carries no permanent physical marker, so dancers can move relatively easily in and out of the potentially stigmatizing role. In this way, belly dance is a *discreditable*, rather than *discredited* stigma (Goffman 1963). In other words, the stigmatizing attribute is invisible and not widely known, but could be damaging if its presence is discovered.

People are stigmatized when they are devalued as a result of being associated with a negative stereotype. Erotic dancers do not have positive reputations in mainstream American culture. This is partly because the public believes erotic dance is not an acceptable way to earn money and judges erotic dance as a violation of morals regarding public nudity (Thompson *et al.* 2003). Also, erotic dancers are marginalized because they challenge norms of female sexuality, such as displaying impersonal sexuality in public without emotional ties (Salutin 1971). Because belly dance is viewed by some members of the public as an erotic performance, dancers may be negatively evaluated as having "unnatural passions" or "blemishes in their moral character" (Goffman 1963:4). This may be especially true for belly dancers given that the vast majority of them do not depend on the activity for their livelihoods. That belly dancers don't rely on the dance for their sole income may heighten judgments of immorality. They have the option to quit the activity, but many choose not to. Instead, they manage annoying comments, strained interactions, odd looks, and snubs using a variety of techniques (Kraus 2010b).

Many dancers with whom I have spoken throughout this project commented on the perception that belly dancers are erotic dancers without my lead. That they shared this belief without prompt suggests that the link between belly dance and erotic dance is a prominent issue for many dancers. For example, Alexandra recalls dancing at an event some people boycotted. "Belly dance has a negative image with sex and prostitution," Alexandra tells me. "We were at a city park and there were people from some church with signs saying that lust is one of the seven deadly sins," Alexandra remembers.

Because some members of the public think belly dancers are erotic dancers, a few dancers have been denied opportunities to perform. Maggie performed a few dances at a coffee house and was asked to stop. Afterwards, she asked the employee for an explanation. She was told her dancing was "inappropriate for the atmosphere." Maggie interpreted the employee's response as an example of how some people believe belly dancers are erotic dancers. "I was honestly really surprised because I try very hard to represent this art form as respectfully as possible," Maggie tells me. "It's really important to me to try, the best I can, to break the negative stereotypes Americans tend to have about belly dancing." Unfortunately, this experience is not uncommon. "This is a problem I have occasionally run into," Maggie confides.

Examining stigma is meaningful partly because it has real consequences for people's involvement in an activity. Despite many benefits, dirty looks, rude or judgmental comments, and snubs can negatively affect participation in leisure

(Jones 2000). While Maggie's dancing in the coffee shop was cut short due to negative interpretations of the dance, some people delay entering the world of belly dance due to similar unfavorable perceptions.

Now in her fifties, Paige contemplated getting involved in belly dance for almost ten years before she registered for lessons. "Why did it take you so long?" I ask. "The image that belly dancers are strippers has always been there, and it is one reason I held back from taking classes," Paige tells me. Like many members of the general public, Paige was unaware of different belly dance styles. When she found a style of belly dance that appealed to her that she felt was distinct from erotic dance, she became more comfortable with getting involved. "I went to one of the performances, and they had a folkloric presentation, and I fell in love with it. They were dressed in the Turkish gypsy style, covered stomachs, and peasant looking clothes, and I really liked that," Paige remembers. In fact, many dancers use various styles of dance and costuming to influence how they are perceived.

"Our troupe portrays it in a quality way"

Like swimmers who attempt to present their body as a non-sexual machine (Scott 2010), some belly dancers engage in several body management strategies to avoid being an object of a sexualized gaze. They manipulate their personal fronts to manage how their dancing is perceived. A front consists of bodily movements, facial expressions, clothing, and hairstyles, which are used to control the impression people give to others (Goffman 1959; Hughes 2000). Some belly dancers practice different styles of dance and pay careful attention to how they execute movements to help minimize the extent to which they are likened to erotic dancers. In fact, some troupes have guidelines for the costumes that dancers wear at performances which generally conform to standard American notions of beauty. Embracing the values of a dominant culture illustrates what Ezzell (2009) calls "normative identification." When belly dancers attempt to conform to accepted notions of feminine beauty, they uphold standard ideas of attractiveness. For instance, Rose's troupe selects "tasteful" makeup and visually appealing clothing. They do not want to appear frightening or scary, so they avoid being dramatic or dark in ways that may stray too far from stereotypical guidelines for American beauty. According to Rose, an attractive appearance helps enhance the image of belly dance. Rose explains:

> I think we have brought [belly dance] to a new light, and I think [the general public] is more accepting of it . . . I hope that is because of the way our troupe portrays it in a quality way instead of in an unquality way, such as unacceptable clothing . . . Yes, of course your stomach is going to show in belly dancing, but

it is tastefully done with tasteful makeup. Everything is not too over the top or too theatrical. We do put on heavy makeup, but we do try to look more refined.

Rose's comments mirror how some women avoid the "Tami Bakker look" with their makeup (Beausoleil 1994).

Similar to Rose's group, Tabitha wears what she refers to as modest costumes. Tabitha used to dance in restaurants in the large metropolitan city where she lived prior to her current place of residence. "I'm a little more conservative in my dress," Tabitha tells me. When Tabitha performed, she wore "the traditional tube dress, whereas a lot of the girls wore skimpy costumes," she tells me. Tabitha prefers to dress more conservatively while dancing because she works for a university. "Heaven forbid someone sees this and goes 'Oh, that's my teacher'" – a comment echoing my concerns when I danced while in graduate school. "What's problematic with somebody recognizing you as their teacher?" I inquire. Without hesitation, she replies, "Because they might interpret it to be like a strip form. It's just not. It's a misinterpretation of what I am trying to communicate to them."

In addition to dress, various accessories are used to minimize the likelihood of sexualizing the body. For example, swimmers adorn their bodies with flippers, goggles, floats, and other devices that function to desexualize the body (Scott 2010). Similarly, some belly dancers verbally communicate that the coin belts that are iconic symbols of belly dance and standard costume pieces represent a very old custom of people wearing coins on their bodies. Although coin belts emphasize parts of the body that are historically associated with femininity and could be deemed sexual, attaching a historically utilitarian purpose to the costume works to prevent the dance from being defined as sexual.

Along with dress and accessories, behavior is another component of our personal fronts. Dancers monitor their conduct while wearing belly dance costumes. For instance, members of one group sign a contract promising not to drink, smoke, curse, or engage in public displays of affection while in costume, which they believe will help distinguish them from erotic dancers. For instance, Larissa tells me about a time when members of her group danced in a bar while wearing their belly dance costumes. In her twenties, Larissa "flirted with her husband and some other group members danced in sexually suggestive ways," she explains. However, this behavior was not appreciated by other group members. Larissa has since refrained from kissing her husband in public while wearing a belly dance costume. About why behaving in sexually suggestive ways while wearing a belly dance outfit may be problematic, Larissa says, "Because when you are . . . suggestively dancing with your husband, [onlookers] don't know he is your husband. They could think he is some guy you are grinding on. They are going to be like, 'That belly dancer is doing that [for him], so this belly dancer is going to do that for me,'" she explains. "You have to remember you are representing a culture, and you have to act a little better ... people already have a bad image of belly dancers ... So we try to stay away from that by presenting the more positive things. We are very covered and very modest. We are not cussing, we are not drinking, and we are not doing all kinds of horrible things."

In addition to managing their personal front with makeup, costumes, and behavior while in belly dance attire, dancers also make extensive use of "body work" (Hochschild 1979). In this case, body work refers to movement execution and tip-taking practices in order to manage emotions. One way dancers try to distinguish belly dance from erotic dance is to maintain a certain posture. Because many belly dance moves are executed using the hips and stomach, it is easy for a dancer to release her back and display her protruding buttocks. During one belly dance class I observe, the instructor reminds the students to keep their "booties tucked" because "we must protect our reputation as belly dancers." The instructor suggests dancing with one's backside sticking out is not acceptable within belly dance and may encourage an erotic gaze.

Likewise, Brooke, who has taught belly dance for decades, instructs her students not to "do any kind of pelvic forward movements." Rather, "all of their movements are pelvic to the back." Furthermore, she distinguishes between a shoulder shimmy (rapidly moving the shoulders back and forth) and a breast shimmy (shaking one's breasts). In addition to carefully executing pelvic and shoulder movements, "We don't do any kind of bump and grind. Our feet are together. If our feet are apart, we are very careful how we are presenting it and what direction we are presenting it." For instance, if Brooke's students perform floor work, their knees point to the side rather than facing the audience. All of these strategies are Brooke's attempt to minimize her and her students' dancing as sexual.

Whether and how one accepts tips is another way some belly dancers engage in body work and manage their personal fronts. Tipping is a common activity, but its meaning varies by the setting and people involved. For example, tipping in America is expected with some service providers, such as wait staff and valets. Tipping is not expected in other contexts, such as in a theater or a college classroom. Tipping dancers is customary and a sign of appreciation in the Middle East (van Nieuwkerk 1995). Traditionally, tipping begins with a "money shower," during which the tipper flings bills (not coins) at the dancer. At some restaurants or parties, someone associated with the establishment or event will initiate a money shower to set the expectation of tipping. However, some American dancers believe that tipping encourages the perception that they are erotic dancers. Furthermore, accepting tips may be more common with some forms of belly dance and in particular contexts compared to others. For instance, tipping is more likely to occur when dancers perform Middle

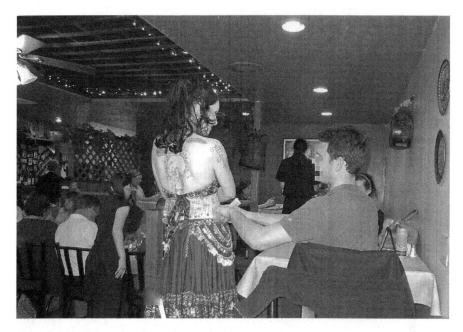

Figure 8.3 Dancer performing and accepting tips at a restaurant

Eastern styles in restaurants (see Figure 8.3). Informal street performances also tend to encourage tipping.

Tipping is one of the most significant ways customers show satisfaction with an erotic dancer's performance (Pasko 2002). Therefore, not accepting tips is one strategy some belly dancers employ to avoid being viewed as erotic dancers. Penelope says, "That is a misperception a lot of people have, and if you go around letting people shove dollar bills in your belt . . . that's what strippers do." Likewise, Julia says, "It is about not going to a restaurant and letting people tuck dollars down my skirt." While some belly dancers do not accept tips, others have rules for how they receive tips, which also function to distant belly dance from erotic dance. Some dancers allow tips being placed in their wrist band, in the back or side of a hip belt, or left in a jar. Other dancers collect tips in baskets they carry on their head or in tambourines. Whether and how someone accepts tips reflects strategies that some dancers use to separate themselves from erotic dancers.

Dressing in particular ways, strategically moving the body, and tip-taking management are all techniques dancers use to define a belly dance performance as non-sexual and control how audiences perceive the dancers. Likewise, in her research on swimmers, Scott (2010) demonstrates how swimmers use their bodies not only to "look good," but to uphold general rules that public swimming is not a sexual activity despite being "near naked."

"I don't want to cross that line"

Some dancers distance themselves from erotic dancers or those belly dancers whom they believe could be linked to erotic dancers. A few belly dancers have refused direct requests from erotic dancers to teach them some belly dance moves because they do not want belly dance and erotic dance to be performed in the same setting. Similarly, Julia distances herself from dancers whom she thinks could promote an association between belly dance and erotic dance. As Julia explains:

> I'm not the modesty police of belly dancers. I'm perfectly OK with people showing as much of their body as they want, but I do think, especially at family-friendly events, you really have to be respectful of how other people perceive you. You have to put some space between yourself and your audience and not shake your butt in the husband's face when his wife is sitting next to him or his kids are right there or wearing a short skirt . . . Dropping and spreading your knees open when you're on stage at eye level. Things like that that I've seen people do.

Julia touches on several aspects of some belly dance that she believes encourages the perception that belly dancers are erotic dancers. She continues to tell me about an event at which belly dancers and dancers from a local gentlemen's club performed. After the belly dancers finished their performance, they joined the dancers from the gentlemen's club by dancing in a large window. But Julia did not approve of this behavior. "I don't care if you're a stripper . . . You make your money however you want to. But the rest of us are trying to say we are not strippers. We are family-friendly. This is appropriate for all ages and for all people, and then you go and dance right next to the strippers and that kind of sends mixed messages." Julia creates boundaries between her dance and other forms of entertainment by emphasizing that belly dance is "family-friendly."

Belly dance has an on and off relationship with burlesque. As I mentioned in Chapter 1, belly dance was associated with burlesque houses when it was first popularized in the United States. Similar to Julia's concern with being associated with erotic dancers, Grace attempts to distance herself from burlesque dance. Throughout her thirty years of involvement in belly dance, Grace has been asked to join burlesque performances. However, Grace is not comfortable participating in burlesque shows, because she works to keep burlesque and belly dance separate. Several dancers in Grace's troupe participate in burlesque, and they have occasionally asked Grace to join them. "I don't want to cross that line because I've had this fine line for years. I don't want to go there, and now you're saying let's cross that line. We've been fighting for years against that." Like Grace's attempt to distance herself from some of her group members' burlesque activities, some affiliates of potentially discredited groups will separate themselves from those within their group whom they feel encourage negative perceptions. For instance, "stripteasers" use a process called "resistance" to distance themselves from dancers they think are "sleazy" (Ronai and Cross 1998).

"I don't want to put it out there"

Some marginalized people engage in secrecy by separating their lives between groups of people who are aware of the potentially stigmatizing characteristic and others from whom the discredited trait is hidden (Goffman 1963; Thompson et al. 2003). The concern with some people learning about their involvement in belly dance is that a dancer's relationship with those people and/or perceptions they have of dancers will be negatively affected. Belly dancers may risk a loss of status or money associated with employment opportunities.

Similar to other marginalized groups (Goffman 1963), belly dancers divide their social world into people they tell about their participation in the dance and those from whom they keep their dancing a secret. Like other people who keep their involvement in discredited activities hidden from their acquaintances (see Thompson and Harred 1992), some belly dancers primarily disclose their involvement to their family and close friends. However, some are apprehensive about telling co-workers and people at religious organizations about their involvement. Many dancers are highly educated and have active professional careers, such as teaching, science, business, and counseling. Just as I was concerned with how my dissertation committee, students, and potential future colleagues may perceive my involvement in belly dance, some dancers ponder how their clients, co-workers, and bosses may evaluate them if they brought much of their belly dance identity into the workplace. For example, even after fifteen years of participating in the belly dance scene, Sabrina does not tell many of her co-workers about her involvement in belly dance because she is concerned about their perception of her. Her boss, with whom she is close at work, is one exception. Sabrina explains that:

> A majority of people are not familiar with belly dance. I'm afraid they might have the wrong idea. I prefer not to tell [people] at work. My boss knows, because I have a close professional relationship with him, so I thought it was OK. But, [I don't tell] everyone. People might … have a different opinion of you [and think] you're a dirty girl because you dress like that and expose your belly.

Lilly was involved in belly dance for less than five years. When we first met she was in her twenties and working on her doctorate degree in a business related field. Most of her colleagues were men and "the environment is very professional," Lilly tells me. Lilly wonders if "maybe my colleagues would think I'm a stripper" if she disclosed her involvement in belly dance to them. She feels she can "only reveal this part of me to close friends." In fact, by the second time we converse, Lilly has graduated, is working full time at a university, and no longer participates in belly dance partly due to these concerns about how her involvement would be viewed by other professionals in her field and by her students. "Other than graduating, what happened that you stopped dancing?" I ask her. "It was that part of me that felt it would be embarrassing in front of my students," Lilly replies. "As I was getting tenure, my boss had an issue with women in general, and he had an issue with my age. I didn't want to give him anything more to look unprofessional," Lilly continues.

Along with not freely disclosing their involvement in belly dance to people at their places of employment, some dancers do not share their participation with people in their religious congregations. Although belly dance can be a source of spirituality for some dancers and that spirituality occasionally overlaps with organized religious practices (Kraus 2010a), dancers sometimes fear that there would be repercussions if some of their fellow church-goers discover they belly dance.

Christian groups, to varying degrees, emphasize male leadership, female modesty, and approved sexual behavior within marriage (Flory 1996, 2000; Roof and McKinney 1987; Steensland et al. 2000). Christian women are highly valued for their caregiving and sexual purity (Ammerman 1987; Christ 1987; McGuire 2008; Raphael 2008; Woodhead 2002). Furthermore, conservative, and to some extent, moderate mainline Protestants – more so than other Christians – prohibit dancing and wearing revealing clothing, such as short skirts, sheer garments, low necklines, and tops that reveal the stomach (Roof and McKinney 1987; Steensland et al. 2000). These more conservative and moderate groups may also limit music and dance to songs deemed appropriate for church (Flory 1996, 2000; McGuire 2008). Because it may be considered sexually suggestive and a distraction, dance is viewed with contempt in some Western religions (Stewart 2000), so some belly dancers hesitate to share their involvement in belly dance with people at their houses of worship.

One of Shelby's friends suggested she belly dance in her church talent show that occurs annually at the end of every Sunday school year. But, Shelby hesitates. "Why wouldn't the church be ready for it?" I ask. "Well, depending on the costume," Shelby replies. "Some of the older members of the church already have issues with me. If I come in wearing a belly dancing outfit, then they'd really have issue with me," she continues. Shelby explains that her church has gone through a lot of changes, such as updating their music. "We have members who are just not happy about change. Belly dancing would be a big change," Shelby tells me. Shelby recalls some people at her church objecting

154

to a liturgical dance, which primarily consisted of ballet moves. She adds, "The costumes I think they would have trouble with, and just with a lot of people, so many people associate belly dancing with being sexual."

"I am a Middle Eastern dancer"

Participants and scholars alike sometimes struggle with what to call this dance. I write a letter of endorsement for a colleague who conducts similar research and is being evaluated for a promotion. We debate whether to refer to this activity as belly dance based on the perception that some of her reviewers may have of this label. Rather than using belly dance in her letter, I use phrases such as Middle Eastern dance and women who participate in Middle Eastern dance. The name we give a phenomenon influences its meaning and how people react to it (Atkins-Sayre 2005). Pedophiles refer to themselves as "boy lovers" (Durkin and Bryant 1999), garbage collectors are "sanitation engineers" (Thompson and Harred 1992), and "fat" men are "cuddly bears" (Monaghan 2005). Similarly, some belly dancers use "semantic manipulation" (Durkin and Bryant 1999) by referring to belly dance as "Middle Eastern" dance.

If an activity can be linked to art or culture, it appears more legitimate (Hughes 2000). For instance, Fawn uses the term "Middle Eastern" dance because she considers it more accurate than belly dance. Fawn explains, "[Calling the dance Middle Eastern] takes it up to the level of authenticity. Belly dance is a misnomer. There's a lot more than just the belly."

Using alternative speech increases an activity's prestige and reduces negative images associated with it (Durkin and Bryant 1999; Thompson and Harred 1992). Because it sounds more legitimate and credible, saying "Middle Eastern" dance can help dancers avoid awkward inquiries. Ophelia tells me about an uncomfortable interaction with one of her colleagues. "You belly dance? They have a studio for this?" her co-worker asks. "This is exactly the conversation I am too exhausted to have today," Ophelia recalls. "When I talk to people like that, I prefer to say Middle Eastern dancing because . . . I don't have to get into the whole conversation." Ophelia partly uses the term "Middle Eastern" dance because it helps her avoid confrontations and allows her to refrain from justifying her participation in the activity.

Legitimation techniques, including semantic manipulation, are likely used when an activity lacks a unified symbolic meaning and public approval (Irwin 2001). The meaning of belly dance is ambiguous. It walks a fine line between appropriate and inappropriate sexuality, which can vary depending on the context in which one dances. Because belly dance taps into issues of the body and sexuality, and there is a great deal of ambiguity surrounding sexuality in America (Barkan 2004), dancers attempt to legitimize the dance.

"I try to figure out if it's a good time for a feminist intervention"

Education is a final technique dancers use to confront negative stereotypes and change perceptions that belly dance is the same as erotic dance. They use public performances as avenues to share what belly dance "really" is. These dancers hope that if people see a good performance and learn about belly dance, their perceptions of it may change, thereby enhancing its legitimacy. Highlighting positive aspects of belly dance is similar to how other groups attempt to "upgrade" (Salutin 1971) their tainted activities by suggesting they are valuable and useful (Thompson and Harred 1992). For instance, "fat" men claim they enjoy being larger, rather than associate obesity with sickness or disease (Monaghan 2005). Many belly dancers enjoy educating the public. Bailey remarks, "What I like about performing is to show people the beauty of belly dance. I think there are a lot of misconceptions about exactly what belly dancing is. A lot of people have a . . . bad idea about it and that you are akin to a stripper."

Similar to Bailey, Tiffany attempts to educate the public during some belly dance shows she hosts. "I try to figure out if it's a good time for a feminist intervention," Tiffany comments. These opportunities typically occur when she runs the show and has the time to talk with audiences about the dance. "I like to joke about how we're wearing more clothing than the audience, by volume or by weight, even though we happen to be showing our bellies. This gets people to realize that our costumes are actually quite modest, and thus not geared toward seduction," Tiffany explains. Furthermore, Tiffany sometimes shares the history of belly dance and "jokes how if someone had an image of a sultry scantily-clad siren prancing through a harem, they should forget it, because that's totally not what belly dance is about." Tiffany also likes to "emphasize that belly dance is family-friendly and how in many of its original cultural contexts, it's a folk dance in the sense that it's done by large swaths of the population, from kids to old folks." In these ways, Tiffany strategically defines belly dance for the audience in an attempt to frame how her and other dancers are viewed. Like Julia's earlier comments, labeling belly dance as "family-friendly" creates symbolic boundaries around her form of dance and by doing so, suggests that other forms of dance may not be.

Being a male dancer in a woman's world

While many female belly dancers negotiate perceptions that they are erotic dancers, male dancers manage a different public image. Because belly dance is dominated by women, men who participate in this activity may be viewed with suspicion. Some people may be uncomfortable with male dancers partly because it makes visible the invisible power structures. A veiled status represents power and privilege, so when men's dancing bodies are displayed, they are no longer hidden and free from scrutiny (McKay *et al.* 2005). Therefore, male dancing threatens masculinity by drawing attention to invisible power (Burt 2009). Traditional masculinity is expected to be active, so it is considered problematic for a male body to be the passive subject of a gaze and desired (Buchbinder 2013; McKay *et al.* 2005). In contrast, it is more acceptable to display the female body because it is assumed to be intended for male heterosexual consumption (Buchbinder 2013).

Similar to men in female-dominated professions who sometimes encounter negative stereotypes from those who are not involved in their career (see Williams 1992), male dancers occasionally experience or imagine negative views from outsiders. There are huge risks if males fail to conform to hegemonic ideals of manhood, such as a diminished sense of self, losing friends, and being teased (Kimmel 2008). Andy tells me about a time he danced lunch shows at a bar that caters to bikers and truckers. Although he was booked specifically for ladies' events, occasionally male patrons would enter. "There were a couple of derogatory remarks, and then I would pull out an eight foot python, and it's OK," Andy tells me. Onlookers act like "gender police" by judging whether our behavior meets accepted standards of gender performance. Men who don't measure up to hegemonic ideals are considered sub-par and risk being reprimanded and labeled gay, effeminate, or wimpy (Connell 2002). Some of the male patrons at the bar attempted to sanction Andy's dancing by making fun of him. Performing exaggerated notions of masculinity by incorporating a snake into his dance helped quieten some public objections to Andy's dancing.

Denny "gets crap all of the time" for his involvement in belly dance. "There is a giant misconception of male belly dancers. A lot of Americans see it as a female thing," Denny says. But Denny doesn't agree with that perception. "With everything and every walk in life, there is always a male counterpart," Denny explains. Although he fields comments from various family members about his participation in the dance, his mother is "very happy I am dedicated, but I have shown her a few dances, and sometimes she thinks they are too lewd and too creepy, and sometimes I look like a goofball," Denny laughs.

Along with his family, Denny's friends also have differing opinions of his participation in belly dance. "Some of my friends think it is the neatest thing in the world . . . They ask me all of these questions," Denny says of his supportive peers. At the same time, he has other friends who "laugh at me." Denny claims that the unsupportive comments and jabs do not bother him. "I just let it roll off my back because one of these days you will get into a situation where you are the token something and there is going to be misconceptions. I am not going to force it on people, but if they want to know, I am going to explain

157

to them how big of a role the male is in belly dancing," Denny continues. Therefore, similar to some female dancers, Denny uses education to counteract perceptions of men in belly dance.

Furthermore, letting comments "roll off his back" requires Denny to engage in "emotion work" (Hochschild 1979). Discredited people, not those they encounter, perform most of the work needed to maintain smooth inter-actions (Cahill and Eggleston 1995). Many of the strategies identified in this chapter are forms of emotion work, such as using semantic manipulation as a cognitive attempt to change images of belly dance. Furthermore, belly dancers need to manage their own emotions, such as anger and frustration. Utilizing stigma management techniques may help minimize unfavorable perceptions of belly dance, thereby helping dancers manage their feelings about unflatter-ing public attitudes.

Similar to Denny, Phil also engages in some emotion work to manage nega-tive perceptions of him being a male dancer. When Phil first started belly dance, his biggest concern was that he would be considered a novelty act. "I call it the lizard boy syndrome," Phil begins. The lizard boy is a side show act at the circus. "No one pays attention to the fact that he studied at Julliard or can play the violin or the piano. He's the lizard boy and that's it," Phil con-tinues. Making the comparison with belly dance, Phil says, "Everyone focuses on the fact that you are male." In this way, Phil, and other male belly dancers, lose their social privilege of invisibility. They stand out in a sea of women. Phil did not want to be valued solely for being a male dancer. He wants his skills and talents to be appreciated beyond the fact that he is male.

Phil recalls one performance after which someone said to him, "For a guy you dance really well . . . For a guy!" Phil exclaims. "The ultimate vengeance is being invited back places because people love what you did or women com-ing after me saying 'I've never seen a man dance, and I'm happy to see you dance because that was amazing,'" Phil tells me. Recently, Phil performed at one event and the host told him that he was an inspiration to at least one male who attended his performance. After seeing Phil dance, this man began taking regular belly dance classes with the instructor who hosted the event. "If I can get other people to love belly dance, I can do that." Part of the emotion work that Phil engages in is focusing on the positive comments he receives about his dancing and being an inspirational role model for other male dancers.

Like Phil, Henry also "wants to make some kind of lasting mark." A few years ago, Henry experienced what he refers to as an "interesting transition." For many years, Henry sought out advice from as many different dancers as he could, both male and female. "Every time I would go to a workshop or event, I would ask teachers what advice would you give to a male belly dancer?" Henry remembers. He eventually exhausted all of the feedback he received. However, a few years ago the tables turned and "people started coming to me and asking 'what advice do you have for a male belly dancer?'" Male dancers like Phil and Henry feel a great deal of satisfaction when they reach a point where they are respected as leaders in dance rather than being a "side show" act.

Furthermore, although Henry knows how to drum, he never drums on stage. His concern is that once people see him drum, they automatically assume he is the drummer because being the drummer is the more socially traditional role for a man (it is more stereotypical for women to be seen and men to be heard). Before people know he is a dancer, it is common for Henry to interact with people who assume he is a drummer. When Henry's wife is with him, people typically acknowledge her as the dancer. To ensure that he is first thought of as a dancer, Henry refrains from drumming on stage.

Likewise, Kevin strategically makes decisions whether he will dance at a hafla based on who is in attendance. "If you have a lot of people who are from the local manufacturing plant . . . [my dancing] might detract from them coming to some of the other haflas," Kevin says. Because these gatherings tend to be fundraisers for his group, he does not want to deter potential paying audience members. "What is it about those employees?" I ask. "There's a lot of homophobia in this area. I'm straight, but there are a lot of people who go like 'Oh no stop doing that,' that type of thing." Kevin implies that some people, especially from the local factory, assume he is gay because he is involved in belly dance. "With this type of thing you have to try to find the accepting audience. [His group] are trying to do a lot of good to spread Middle Eastern culture. I don't want to detract from that because it's more about them than it is about me," Kevin explains. Just like jazz and ballet dancers (Mennesson 2009), some male belly dancers confront stereotypes that they are homosexual, which male dancers protest and attempt to avoid.

Similar to some female belly dancers who divide their world into people who know they belly dance and those from whom they keep it a secret, Henry also strategically chooses to whom he discloses his involvement in belly dance, but for very different reasons. Henry keeps "a very strict work–life separation." Henry does not disclose his involvement in dance to his co-workers. Only one or two of his co-workers know he dances, and he does not volunteer any information about it. For instance, when he travels for dance-related activities, such as out of town workshops, Henry does not tell his colleagues why he will be away from work. Henry works in engineering, "a very male-dominated field." He "plays things very conservatively at work." About the people he works with, Henry comments, "some of them are very conservative, so I don't actively advertise for fear that I might cause waves." Therefore, while many female dancers navigate perceptions that they are erotic dancers, many male dancers manage perceptions that men do not belong in belly dance. In doing so, male and female dancers rely on very similar stigma management strategies, but for different reasons.

Renegotiating public perceptions of belly dance

Outsiders using relatively narrow guidelines to judge belly dancers create challenges for those who participate in this social world. When members of the general public, their family, friends, co-workers, and religious adherents look down upon, eroticize, or objectify one's involvement in belly dance, belly dancers have to manage innuendoes, jokes, snubs, and perceptions of the erotic precisely because the activity has a very public component.

Throughout the many years that I have participated in and written about belly dance, I have encountered people attempting to tell me what belly dance "is," which more often than not revolves around sexuality. Some of my colleagues sometimes dismiss belly dancers (or studies of them) because they define the activity as akin to stripping, while others ask me to write or talk about belly dance in ways that exaggerate its sexuality. Just as many dancers engage in reality definition contests (Loseke 1987) with their friends, family, co-workers, and members of the general public, I too have debated with colleagues about the extent to which belly dance is and isn't sexual. In this way, like many other dancers, I also engage in numerous stigma management techniques and reality definition contests even among fellow academics.

The extent to which dancers implement various management strategies within any given setting partly depends on and is constrained by that context. Some techniques, such as ceasing a performance and educating an audience, are not feasible because they break the operating rules of that interaction. Other settings, such as small group interactions or one-on-one conversations, may be more conducive to thorough explanations of how a dancer experiences and defines belly dance. Further still, dancers utilize numerous forms of body work and costuming practices attempting to prevent audiences from defining their dance as overly sexual or erotic.

Likewise, different stigmatizing behavior elicits particular management techniques. Verbal comments about the dance may be best addressed with semantic manipulation and references to the dance being "family-friendly." Physical attempts to redefine the dance, such as avoiding movements that may be deemed too sexual and encouraging patrons to tip within particular guidelines are utilized during actual performances. Many uncomfortable situations may require the dancer to engage in emotion work either during or after an encounter to stifle feelings and help him or her emotionally recover from unpleasant interactions.

Although I have dedicated this chapter and the previous one to a variety of challenges that people experience within belly dance, costs do not always lead to abandonment, but rather to the adoption of perseverance strategies (Lamont et al. 2014). Similar to people who push through the challenges of other leisure activities, such as running (Lamont et al. 2014) and participation in dog sports (Baldwin and Norris 1999), many dancers continue their involvement in dance most likely because, like many other serious leisure pursuits (Stebbins 2011), the benefits are meaningful to a sense of self and outweigh the costs. Rather than completely leaving an activity, leisure participants use strategies that allow them to remain involved (Lamont *et al.* 2014).

One reason why people persevere is because the activity brings opportunities that people would not have outside of it (Lamont *et al.* 2014). I have remained involved in belly dance partly because dancing with my troupe gives me access to art events, renaissance festivals, and other gatherings that I may not otherwise know about. In fact, although it resulted in extremely uncomfortable feelings for me, I attended the evening event I described earlier in this chapter partly because I have never been a part of that kind of setting before, and I doubt I would ever have a similar opportunity if it weren't for my participation in belly dance.

Chapter 9

The finale

I use the case of belly dance to analyze how participants draw on symbolic resources in female-dominated leisure subcultures for the creation of individual and group identities, and the challenges they encounter along the way. I explore how participants use these symbols to mark group membership and to resist some aspects of the mainstream that they find offputting. Because belly dance is highly visible and dancers frequently interact with outsiders, I examine the interplay between participants' views of themselves and how outsiders perceive them.

Examining participation in leisure subcultures is meaningful because involvement in these social worlds influences the everyday lives of participants. Through this study of belly dance, we learn about the role that leisure subcultures play in the lives of adult women and men. This project sheds light on how people spend their free time, how participants do friendships, and the production and presentation of identities. Studying belly dance teaches us about subcultural internal diversity and how subcultural norms can overlap with larger cultural values.

To these ends, I have demonstrated how belly dance provides resources for a wide range of identity work. Both men and women utilize tools, such as costumes and movements, to perform a variety of masculinities and femininities. Participants also use belly dance to reconnect with their bodies and develop more body-positive feelings. For some people, belly dance is a site to explore sensuality and sexuality on their own terms. The gendered and embodied nature of belly dance offers women an opportunity to form close bonds with each other, and structural components of the activity are conducive to a variety of ways that women do same-sex friendships. Along with building friendships, several participants use belly dance as a space to explore the spiritual side of their lives. Finally, participation in leisure activities becomes part of people's sense of self to varying degrees. I illustrate several aspects of the dance that students and teachers use to both construct and confer a belly dance identity. Furthermore, I show how a sense of self outside of leisure and group norms internal to the activity coalesce in the adoption of dance names.

Although belly dance provides many resources for the construction of self and social relationships, identity work within this leisure subculture is not without its challenges. Although dancers find friendship, self-expression, and body-positive messages inside of belly dance circles, they also confront status hierarchies, power differentials, and conflict surrounding authentic participation in this social world. Furthermore, because belly dancers frequently interact with the general public, dancers navigate (real or imagined) disconnects between how they view themselves and how outsiders evaluate them.

Without question there are many aspects of belly dance not covered here. The Middle Eastern and North African (among others) cultural systems surrounding belly dance are much more extensive than I have explored. I have also not given much attention to issues of orientalism and acculturation beyond debates of authenticity and legitimacy. Similarly, except for my discussion of men's historical involvement in the dance, I do not delve deeply into the historical and political culture that frames the history of Middle Eastern dance. Furthermore, I do not extensively pursue issues of sexual orientation that no doubt shape some questions particularly related to male belly dancers. Intriguing topics, such as psychological consequences and objective measures of health also fall outside of the scope of this book, as do interesting issues related to race, nationality, and social class. At least in the areas I observed, there is a dearth of racial variation in belly dance, especially given the cultural roots of this dance form. As one dancer comments, "there is an absence of our black sisters." All of these topics merit further investigation.

Leisure as a break

Although there is a professional counterpart to belly dance, and a few of the people in this study made or make their livings through belly dance, the activity is a form of leisure for the vast majority of dancers in the United States. Leisure pursuits provide both men and women with a space to take a break from their regular lives. For women in particular, leisure offers an opportunity to leave their caretaking roles (Dilley and Scraton, 2010; Stalp *et al.* 2008). At a micro level, belly dance is an activity women enjoy to care for themselves without focusing on their other responsibilities, such as family or work (Moe 2012). It provides a break from everyday chores, errands, and concerns. In belly dance, participants navigate gender, construct spiritual experiences, build friendships, find acceptance of body diversity, and experience belonging to a larger community. Structurally, belly dance provides a refuge from cultural messages regarding ideal appearances and an opportunity for women to spend time with other women.

"Describe a normal day for you," I ask Dena. After Dena wakes up, she feeds her cats, eats breakfast, and sits down at her computer to read e-mail and Facebook posts. She often looks at videos or browses articles related to belly dance styles and occasionally visits Amazon's digital music store. "So it sounds like there is quite a bit of dance-related stuff going on," I observe. "In the mornings, yes. Lots that is, or often is, dance-related," Dena responds. Her afternoons are spent watching television, running errands, and preparing to teach belly dance classes in the evenings, which happens about two or three nights a week. In the evenings she does not teach, Dena watches television along with working on costuming or other craft projects.

"It sounds like a good chunk of your everyday is involved in belly dance. Is belly dance a break away from anything or is it fairly entwined in your everyday life?" I ask. "It certainly started out as a break back when I started," Dena responds. "It served as that a lot when I was working. But, now that I'm not working a day job, belly dance is my job. It's also my passion." Dena explains how the role of belly dance in her life changed since she retired from her legal profession. Now, Dena devotes more time to researching belly dance as she continues to teach as much as she did when she was working. Belly dance remains a place "where any worries I have – financial, health, family, etc. – melt away and only the dance exists," Dena says. Although the dance no longer provides much contrast from her working life, it continues to offer some refuge from everyday concerns.

"I loved playing dress-up when I was little because all of my sisters are all older than me, so I'd play with their prom dresses," Norma comments. She continues, "The costumes are just so much fun. They just make me feel really special when I have them on. Following up on her thoughts about feeling special, I inquire, "What do you mean by feeling special?" "Feeling like I don't just blend into the crowd anymore," Norma replies. When she was a young adult, she felt that she "would have made a wonderful doormat, and I did because people would just walk all over me and forget that I was there. I was very quiet. I would blend into the background no matter where I was, and I don't do that anymore," Norma explains. Especially at her work, "sometimes I like to keep [belly dance] a little secret. I am really conservative at work. I pay a lot of attention to detail. I am extremely anal when it comes to my work." But in dance, she feels "like I can open up and break out and do something fun. It's something so different from the rest of my life," Norma says. Belly dance is unlike Norma's everyday existence because "I am a real nerd," she chuckles because she plays video games and spends a lot of time on her computer.

While finishing this book, I contemplate the extent to which and how belly dance has been a break from my everyday life. Similar to Dena when she first got involved in the activity, belly dance is mostly an escape from my work (although I recognize the irony that presently most of my academic writing revolves around belly dance). In my working life, I have perfectionist tendencies. Of course I fail miserably at perfectionism, but it is an unreasonable benchmark to which I frequently hold myself. Attempting to be perfect is typically the only way I feel "good enough." I have always used belly dance as a place to play and try to let go of that perfectionism and attention to detail. My most enjoyable times in dance are when I get together with other dancers and musicians at drum circles or other casual get-togethers. We don't rehearse for a specific performance, there is very little structure, and we are less concerned about perfecting movements. We simply dance for the enjoyment of music, movement, and company. In this way, I use belly dance to honor a playful, free-spirited, and somewhat spontaneous side of my identity.

Furthermore, as many of us experience at our jobs or in the classroom, I am constantly evaluated in my career. My department reviews all pre-tenured faculty on a yearly basis until they receive tenure. Although this is very helpful for ensuring one is on track to earn tenure and affords opportunities for feedback to enhance one's professional development, the yearly evaluation process can be emotionally challenging. In addition to the yearly pre-tenure assessment, the faculty in my department are evaluated by all of our department colleagues on our productivity in teaching, research, and service. Our merit pay (in the years that we receive it) is heavily based on how our colleagues judge our records and experiences for prior years. Furthermore, I am evaluated every semester by the students in my classes on my course design and teaching effectiveness. In addition, every time I submit a paper to be considered for publication in a journal or a grant application to a funding agency, I am assessed (and the more common decisions in both arenas are to reject submissions). Finally, when I run for leadership positions within professional organizations, I am compared to other candidates and risk not being selected. In sum, I am evaluated and ranked on a fairly regular basis in my professional life. Belly dance is an arena in which I try to escape that critique and judgment. Although I am far from the most talented dancer, my mistakes and flaws are typically forgiven. In this sense, belly dance helps me work on a greater sense of self-acceptance and forgiveness.

Similarly, I use belly dance partly to move into the background and take a break from leadership roles. In fact, my troupe mates joke that I always situate myself in the back of our weekly classes or in workshops (and they are absolutely correct!). As a college professor, I perform and lead every time I teach a class, give a conference presentation, participate in meetings, and serve in professional leadership roles. Since I perform and lead so much in my working life, taking a back seat and letting others lead is a welcome break for me. As a follower, I can relax a little more because I do not have think about which moves I will perform next.

Finally, belly dance is my regular social outlet. Being involved in dance provides some structure for my non-working life. It offers me opportunities to dance, listen to musicians, and attend shows that I may not otherwise. In addition, the meaning that I attach to my experiences within American Tribal Style dancing is one of cooperation and interdependence of dancers. In this sense, one of the greatest benefits that I receive from participating in belly dance is the opportunity to be social and participate in a community. Outside of my work and family, I do not have many social outlets. Although I do not have many close friends within belly dance, it remains one of only a few scenes in my life in which I feel some degree of social connection.

In all of these ways, belly dance is an "activity enclave" that provides a site for identity work that contrasts with my everyday life. Activity enclaves are breaks away from life that provide a safe space for identity negotiation and self-expression (Cohen and Taylor 1992). They allow us to temporarily leave our mundane everyday life and renegotiate identity with a different set of resources than what we may have available to us in our regular existence. We can then take these new resources, renegotiate our sense of self using these resources, and apply them to our everyday lives. In this way, identity is a product of interaction. It is situational and different contexts provide different tools and resources to engage in identity work (Cohen and Taylor 1992).

It is easy to think about belly dance as an activity enclave when we consider some dancers' experiences known as a "con drop" (convention drop) or "event drop." Both of these terms refer to the "down" feeling many dancers face after an intense belly dance convention or multi-day event. The language of "drop" suggests that at least some people experience a "high" during these types of belly dance gatherings. During these events, dancers build or re-establish close connections with people that they rarely see, they are energized by new moves or choreographies, and/or they feel closer to their troupe mates after a successful performance. In sum, there can be a surge of very positive feelings of accomplishment, connection, and excitement that starkly contrast with people's ordinary experiences. Regardless of how happy one is with one's life or how interesting a life one may lead, coming down from such intense experiences can be difficult precisely because they are so different from many people's everyday lives.

Concluding thoughts

Belly dance is a fascinating site for academic exploration because it is a messy social world that contrasts with the grace and elegance of the dance form itself. At least in America, belly dance is overwhelmingly a form of leisure, but it is unique among many other standard leisure activities. As a primarily adult female social world that is rooted in a non-Western culture and revolves around a physical activity, belly dance is qualitatively different from other female-dominated leisure activities, such as quilting, knitting, the Red Hat Society, and others. Belly dance is first and foremost a bodily practice and, as such, provides a layer of complexity that isn't always present in other social worlds and leisure subcultures. As such, dancers manage a range of body issues, including internal norms of body acceptance, cultural notions of beauty, and highly contested expressions of sexuality.

That primarily women participate in belly dance has important gender implications for female as well as male dancers. In some areas, male and female dancers share similar experiences, and in other ways, their experiences are vastly different. Both men and women are attracted to belly dance because it is a dance, which some construct as a creative art form, and an enjoyable way to move their bodies beyond traditional forms of exercise, such as running or working out at a gym. Both male and female dancers operate under similar norms of what characteristics and experiences constitute a belly dancer and both engage in similar dance practices in adopting (or not) a dance name. Furthermore, although the particular perceptions that men and women encounter from outsiders differ, male and female dancers employ similar management strategies to discourage public perceptions that women are inappropriately sexual and men are inappropriately feminine. In addition, although they do so in different ways and to varying degrees, both men and women use belly dance as a site to perform traditional notions of gender. Finally, some men and women infuse the dance with spiritual meaning in comparable ways, such as experiencing flow and building a variety of connections.

At the same time, male and female belly dancers have contrasting experiences that are somewhat anchored in how they perform gender. While some women construct spirituality within belly dance as ties to goddess worship or other women, many men resist these female-centered creations for a combination of the masculine and feminine or they focus on alternative meanings of spirituality altogether. Furthermore, relationships, both positive and negative, are more central to women's experiences compared to men. Although feelings of community are important to them, the male dancers in this study talked very little about friendship. For them, belly dance is overwhelmingly a physical form of exercise and less of a social outlet. On the other hand, the opportunity to build close friendships, especially with other women, is core for women's participation in this social world. For many female dancers, the activity provides a break from either masculine-dominated spaces or areas populated with other women with whom they do not enjoy interacting. On the flip side, women, more so than men, experience strain with other female dancers. Women engage in trash talk, divide themselves into in- and out-groups, and compete with one another for limited resources. Because male and female dancers rarely compete with one another, men, for the most part, are protected from internal conflicts.

Unlike many other leisure activities in the United States, belly dance is rooted in and, to varying degrees, maintains ties to non-Western culture. From these cultures, belly dancers borrow and reimagine a variety of tools, such as names, music, dance, and costumes, which participants use to add a layer of richness and diversity to their lives. That belly dance is rooted in a non-Western culture makes it ripe for controversy surrounding authenticity that taps into power and leadership roles (the ability of teachers and troupe leaders to monitor their students' involvement) and norm disputes (at what point have people deviated so far from these roots that they are no longer considered a belly dancer). Both of these issues have implications for the interpersonal relationships between dancers and they are generally concerns affecting female, more so than male, dancers. Furthermore, connecting to Middle Eastern cultures has various implications for how both male and female dancers do gender and experience their bodies. Some women draw from Middle Eastern and North African standards to support body diversity, while men look to these areas for guidance on appropriate masculine dance.

One of the most intriguing aspects of belly dance for studying social behavior is that it has both an internal culture and a highly visible dimension that is shared with the public. The public performance component of belly dance separates it from many other leisure social worlds and sites of academic inquiry. Not only do belly dancers navigate norms and rules within their world, they must simultaneously manage a variety of interactions with and (sometimes ill-perceived) expectations of the general public. These internal and external values can clash, such as in ideas surrounding the female body and sexuality. Therefore, much of the negotiation that occurs within belly dance involves reality definition contests during which both male and female dancers attempt to define for others their understanding of the dance and their role in it. Some men masculinize the dance in various ways to appease Western notions of masculinity. Some women use body techniques and verbal explanations to distance themselves from presumably more sexualized forms of dance.

Altogether, belly dance sheds light on individual, group, and cultural aspects of human life. At the individual level, we learn about how both males and females construct their identities as men and women within a female-dominated context. Based on the particular style in which one is involved, men work in a multitude of ways and to different degrees to construct traditional notions of masculinity, while women construct varying versions of femininity. Along with gender, participants use a variety of tools within belly dance to construct spiritual experiences, affirm their bodies, and build friendships.

As a role that people play, dancers operate within group-specific norms (both formal and informal) and expectations. Participants constantly balance individual identity work with group expectations. Not everyone plays the role of belly dancer in the same way and there is a lot of room for creating various identities within belly dance. There is some freedom to participate in a role how we wish, but we are not free to do anything we desire. There is a certain amount of restraint that is enforced by people in positions of power. Some conflict stems from debates surrounding authenticity in which some dancers creatively negotiate what constitutes belly dance, while other dancers seek to limit that flexibility. Furthermore, the extent to which dancers abide by group norms results in various rewards, such as performance opportunities and troupe memberships. When dancers do not adhere to norms, there are consequences. Additional internal conflict is rooted in the violation of these generally agreed upon subcultural norms and values.

Finally, at the cultural level, examining belly dance sheds light on how participants negotiate dominant Western ideals regarding masculinity, femininity, body image, and sexuality. Furthermore, we see how those outside messages are balanced with competing internal ideologies. In sum, analyzing belly dance touches on many important theoretical questions including meaning-making, reflexivity, presentation of self, embodiment, and balancing the construction of self with social and cultural norms.

Belly dance is a unique context compared to many other leisure and dance sites. However, many of the patterns discussed within these pages related to multiple aspects of gender, the body, self, and relationships are applicable across a variety of contexts. This transferability of themes that we see inside the world of belly dance to outside of this context suggests a level of robustness and adds further support for many sociological patterns involving leisure subcultures as a site for identity work and the performance of gender.

Appendix: methods

While this book draws from conceptual frames within symbolic interaction, leisure, and other sociological paradigms, the analysis presented here is empirically based in qualitative, ethnographic data utilizing a grounded theory and situational analysis approach. Ethnography is an immersive study of a group, community, and/ or social world. It requires sustained involvement to examine multiple dimensions of group life and the norms and values that members may take for granted. This participation in some slice of social life is typically accompanied by other forms of data, including interviews and questionnaires. Ethnographers utilizing grounded theory typically emphasize processes and the goings on of the settings in which they are located (Charmaz 2014). As an ongoing participant in the community, the story presented here partly draws from my personal experiences in belly dance.

I have been an active member of various belly dance communities since 2002. For the first ten years of my involvement, I took regular classes with a variety of instructors teaching different styles of belly dance (primarily nightclub, tribal fusion, and improvisational tribal style) and occasionally performed in local belly dance shows. In 2012, I joined my first student troupe that was attached to an improvisational tribal style group. With this troupe I performed at local cultural and artistic events. In 2013, I began taking American Tribal Style classes and joined a student troupe later that year. In 2015, I joined the professional ATS troupe with which I currently dance as of the writing of this book. As a student and professional troupe member, I have taken classes, attended numerous practices, participated in workshops, traveled to regional belly dance events, and performed (for pay and voluntarily) in a variety of local and regional public venues. Furthermore, I co-founded (in 2008) and serve as the faculty advisor for my university's belly dance club. Throughout the text, I have offered the reader numerous insights into my experiences, thoughts, and feelings as a full member of the belly dance world.

Ethnographers balance their roles as participants in communities with their research goals. In addition to fully participating, we must keep an analytic eye open and record events and conversations either while they are happening or as soon as we can slip away to write them down. In my case, this meant bringing a notebook to classes, workshops, and performances to record any insights or thoughts I had while the activities were occurring. It also included me returning to my home or hotel room to reflect on what I had observed or experienced in some interaction or at an event. In other words, I constantly balanced my responsibilities as a full participant and my commitment to my various troupes (class, rehearsal, and performance schedules) with my role as a social scientific researcher.

Anderson (2006) calls for ethnographers to disclose any changes in their beliefs or relationships throughout their involvement in the world. In other words, ethnographers demonstrate how they wrestle with issues of membership and participation in these worlds. As I discuss in Chapter 8, I performed at an event that made me highly uncomfortable. At least publicly, most of the other participants did not struggle with the situation as much as I did. In fact, people reported that they quite enjoyed the event, which varies from my own experiences. Furthermore, in Chapter 6, I discuss how my participation and commitment level has grown over the past two years with involvement in my current group. Specifically, I have performed more than I ever have since I entered the world of belly dance (an average of about once a month and more in the summer and fall months) and have acquired more costume pieces than I ever previously owned. As a result, similar to Scott's (2010) experiences with swimming, I have grown increasingly committed to belly dance. This is most likely due to my experiences and interactions with my current instructor and troupe.

Belly dance has always been, and remains, a form of recreation for me. However, as the years have gone on, I have begun to schedule more of my time around my involvement in belly dance. To illustrate, during the summer of 2015, I was mindful of my regular Monday night practice and rehearsals along with various weekend workshops and performances. I scheduled many of my other summer plans during times when they would not conflict with my belly dance related commitments.

My aim throughout this project has been to offer a general understanding of belly dance and the people who engage in this activity utilizing a symbolic interactionist approach with the goal of illuminating several important sociological concepts and patterns. My personal thoughts and experiences have supplemented the data, including interviews, conversations, and observations, rather than serving as a primary focal point. Participating in rehearsals, classes, workshops, performances, and side conversations grants me access to perspectives and experiences that I may not otherwise have that are vital to conducting grounded theory work.

A grounded theory approach

Ethnography involves studying the life of a particular group, so our participation in their world is crucial. Rather than stopping at observation, which occasionally focuses on one aspect of life, ethnography examines a range of activities and interactions within that world (Charmaz 2014). Specifically, grounded theory ethnography aims to understand processes or actions within a setting, not just to describe the setting, providing a more holistic picture of a world and the participants in it (Charmaz 2014).

Grounded theory is historically rooted in American symbolic interactionist sociology in that both grounded theory and symbolic interaction seek to understand our participants' worlds, their beliefs, experiences, and interpretations as best as we can (Charmaz 2014; Clarke 2012). Grounded theory offers a set of "systematic, yet flexible guidelines for collecting and analyzing qualitative data to construct theories from those data" (Charmaz 2014:1). At a general level, the goal of grounded theory is to understand the lives of the people we study and locate their understandings and behavior in a larger social context (Charmaz 2009). These analyses result in situated knowledge about the people we examine (Charmaz 2009).

One hallmark feature of grounded theory is that data collection and analysis are a continuing and cyclical process. Unlike other forms of research, data are examined fairly early in the collection process and new data are gathered based on those examinations (Charmaz 2014; Clarke 2012; Glaser and Strauss 1967). Early analyses inform future data to help flush out potential themes and patterns. Doing so helps us choose participants that provide data for theory construction rather than serving as a representative sample of some population (Glaser and Strauss 1967). This flexibility allows qualitative researchers to follow leads that are suggested by the data that we do not initially anticipate (Charmaz 2014). In this way, data gathering is an iterative process. In fact, much of the material on stigma, some of the work on identity, and a great deal of the discussion of male dancers were gathered late in the analysis and emerge from various conversations, interactions, observations, and experiences I had while writing this book.

Recruitment and data collection

As a full member of the belly dance world, I had an intimate engagement with data gathering. In 2006 and 2007, I visited numerous belly dance classes to introduce myself and the project, and gather names of people interested in this study. I also distributed flyers, posted an announcement on a belly dance community's Internet website and in a statewide belly dance association's newsletter, and attended several public events at which belly dancers were performing and/or present. I introduced myself and the project at these events, obtained names of those interested, and contacted those people.

Furthermore, I asked belly dancers whom I interviewed for names of other dancers who might be interested in participating in this study and contacted some of them. This snowball or chain-referral technique of recruiting participants is standard for qualitative studies (Lofland *et al.* 2006). There may be some concern that asking participants for names of other people potentially interested in the study violates ethics of confidentiality. When I approached potential subjects, I did not tell them who shared their name with me. Also, I did not go back to the subjects who suggested those dancers and tell them who did and did not agree to participate. In a few instances, subjects freely disclosed to one another and other people that they participated in this research. Even in those situations, I did not confirm a subject's involvement in this project.

When talking with dancers about this study, I told them I wanted to learn about the characteristics of people who belly dance, how they became involved in it, and the role it plays in their lives. A few dancers, especially those who had less than six months of belly dance experience, were worried that they did not know enough about belly dance to participate in my research. I told them that I was not interested in how much they know about belly dance, but in their personal experiences with and thoughts about it, which alleviated their concerns.

Partly due to some questionable public perceptions of belly dancers (discussed in Chapter 8), some dancers are suspicious of outsiders' interests in belly dance. In fact, very early on in my recruitment, I attended a yearly gathering and talked with one of the officers of the organization about recruiting participants for this study. She did not know me and was initially suspicious of my intentions. "What do you think we are? Weird?" she defensively asked. She challenged me to "describe your research in five words or less." "I'm interested in who belly dances and why," I responded, which seemed to satisfy her curiosity as she agreed to let me recruit potential subjects at the event. Partially because of suspicions like this, it is helpful that subjects know, or at least be able to trust, me. I wanted subjects to feel comfortable sharing their experiences, which increases data quality and richness. Because I partially recruited through networks in which I already knew dancers, some subjects who did not know me possibly knew other people who could verify my identity. Furthermore, I wanted to maximize the diversity and number of participants in the study to learn about a range of experiences and perspectives. My recruitment efforts between 2006 and 2007 resulted in formal interviews with eighty-one dancers. Seventy-three of the dancers I interviewed lived in the Midwest. Six of the dancers lived in the south. One dancer lived on the east coast, and another dancer resided on the west coast.

In the fall of 2011, I followed up with my participants to learn more about their experiences with belly dance and the extent to which they remained involved in the activity. To contact dancers, I sent emails and notices through social media sites. This process resulted in second interviews with thirty-five dancers. Unfortunately, I was not able to formally interview everyone a second time. After five years, some dancers had moved, and their contact information changed. Furthermore, sadly, a few of them passed away. Toward the end of the project, I added two interviews with male dancers particularly to explore some themes related to gender. These dancers live in the north and on the east coast. Throughout the formal interview process, I remained involved in belly dance, receiving instruction, performing to varying degrees, and attending events, which aided my ethnographic data collection. Along with formal interviews, I draw from countless informal conversations, interactions, and observations across various classes, workshops, festivals, car rides, phone calls, social media discussions, and performances.

During recruitment for the formal interviews, I sampled beyond theoretical saturation, which is a customary sampling criteria for qualitative research (Glaser and Strauss 1967). I attempted to locate and interview dancers until new data ceased to spark original theoretical ideas, categories, or properties most pertinent to the aim of this research. According to Charmaz (2014:213), saturation also means that researchers "defined, checked, and explained relationships between categories and the range of variation within and between your categories" (Charmaz 2014:213). In other words, talking to additional people would not yield new theoretical categories, properties of those categories, relationships between categories, or patterns of variation between categories that are germane to the research topic. Early in my research, I first sought to obtain a variety of experiences from dancers of different ages, years of involvement, and dance styles. Later in my research, I relied on theoretical sampling (Charmaz 2014; Glaser and Strauss 1967) to talk with people about particular ideas that emerged as theoretically relevant (Clarke 2012). I ceased sampling when I believed I had more than sufficient data to illustrate the primary themes and patterns central to the aims of this project.

Developing rapport and the interview process

Developing rapport follows Blumer's (1969) call to respect our subjects and preserve their dignity. We attempt to see the world through their eyes and understand their perspectives, even if we do not personally agree with them. One of the best examples in this research is my work on spirituality and belly dance. In Chapter 5, I describe the one time I experienced spirituality within belly dance. Despite the fact that I would like it to be more spiritual, the dance does not hold much spiritual meaning for me. However, this does not stop me from respecting and working to understand those dancers for whom belly dance is spiritual. My task as a researcher is to understand how they interpret and construct the dance even if my personal experiences differ.

I attempted to establish rapport with dancers in several ways. I disclosed my own involvement in belly dance, how long I've been involved in it, and my various instructors (in the cases where participants know my current and/or former instructors and I thought it would increase his/her comfort level with me). I typically began conversations with friendly, non-threatening small talk. I also talked with several people with whom I have a longstanding relationship in the world of belly dance. Our pre-existing connections no doubt helped with building rapport and increasing comfort levels.

I used a brief survey and semi-structured interviews to collect data from those dancers willing to participate in this study. I first gave dancers a short questionnaire, which primarily consisted of questions about their personal backgrounds and experiences within belly dance, such as how long people have been involved in the dance and dance style preference. The surveys also asked for basic demographic information, such as age, income, education, religious affiliation, and occupation.

After respondents answered the survey questions, I engaged in intensive interviewing, which allows for an in-depth exploration of topics. I began with an interview guide consisting of broad, open-ended questions and topics designed to elicit lengthy and detailed responses, such as how people get involved in belly dance, what they enjoy about belly dance, any challenges they experience with belly dance, and how belly dance fits in with the rest of their lives. Similar topics were covered across interviews, but the order in which questions were discussed varied depending on the flow of the conversation. In this way, the interviews were more like guided conversations (Lofland and Lofland 1995). Although I had an interview guide with open-ended questions and topics for inquiry at some point during our talk, I also remained open to new topics emerging that were meaningful to the dancers. The open-ended nature of the talks allowed me to further explore particularly interesting statements or topics and bypass those that weren't particularly relevant to a respondent (Charmaz 2014).

Both grounded theory and intensive interviewing are flexible and directed, guided and emergent, and paced with room to explore (Charmaz 2014). During the interviews, I invited people to elaborate on their responses and provide examples of some of their answers. Because I am interested in dancers' experiences, I rarely provided them with definitions of concepts that I was investigating as part of the study. For instance, I did not define what I mean by belly dance and what forms of dance are included in this descriptor. I also did not provide dancers with a set definition of spirituality. Refraining from offering definitions of concepts allows dancers to share their own perceptions and various meanings of concepts.

The interviews were conducted in person or by phone and ranged from thirty minutes to over two hours, with an average interview lasting around one hour. Conversations were recorded with dancers' permission and transcribed verbatim. Charmaz (2014) argues that coding full interview transcripts helps safeguard against missing important ideas and helps develop a deeper understanding of the world from which the data are drawn.

Taking into account original interviews and re-interviews, I conducted a total of 128 formal interviews. These participants represent more than fifteen distinct, yet (in some cases) overlapping belly dance communities. To limit the possibility of only interviewing dancers who share similar experiences, I entered the world of belly dance through multiple points by talking with people in different communities. A community is typically a troupe or one instructor and her students. I talked with members of different communities, across a variety of cities and states, and a few dancers located in various regions of the country.

In most cases, the interviews discussed in this book are pooled and treated as one large collection rather than longitudinal data that examines change over time. However, at various points I refer to how a particular dancer's involvement in belly dance changed between our first and second conversation when it was particularly meaningful. In most cases, these discussions revolve around why some former participants eventually left the world of belly dance.

The dancers

Table 1 provides a summary of demographic characteristics gathered during the first set of formal interviews. The vast majority of belly dancers in the United States are women, and the gender composition of the sample reflects this pattern. The participants' involvement with belly dance ranges from one month to over thirty-five years, but most dancers have been involved in belly dance less than ten years at the time of the first interview (several of them are still involved in dance as of the writing of this book). The dancers' ages range from the late teens to the sixties, although most of them are in their twenties and thirties (when ages are mentioned in the text, they mostly refer to dancers' ages during the first wave of data collection). The subjects' education levels range from some college to graduate school, and most dancers have at least a Bachelor's degree. The vast majority of the dancers identify as Caucasian or white. A few are African-American, American Indian, or Indian. The dancers' average annual household incomes range from $20,000 to over $100,000, and most live in households earning at least $35,000 a year. Almost half of the sample is married, and almost half of the sample has been divorced. Almost half of the sample affiliates with a Christian religion, while a third of the sample claims no religious affiliation.

Table 1 *Description of formal interviewees from 2006–2007*

Gender	Female	75 (92%)
	Male	6 (7%)
Age	18–29	28 (35%)
	30–39	20 (25%)
	40–49	15 (19%)
	50–59	11 (14%)
	60 and over	5 (6%)
Relationship	Single	22 (28%)
	In a relationship, but not living with a partner	10 (13%)
	Cohabitating	7 (9%)
	Married	38 (48%)
	Other (separated, engaged)	3 (4%)
	Divorced (yes)	35 (43%)
Race	White	69 (85%)
	African-American	2 (2%)
	Hispanic	2 (2%)
	Other (Asian, Puerto Rican, Amer. Indian)	8 (10%)
Education	Some college	20 (25%)
	Associate's degree	7 (9%)
	Bachelor's degree	17 (21%)
	Some graduate or professional training	12 (15%)
	Graduate or professional degree	25 (31%)
Household income	$10,000 a year or less	6 (8%)
	$10,001–$20,000	6 (8%)
	$20,001–$35,000	19 (25%)
	$35,001–$50,000	12 (16%)
	$50,001–$100,000	26 (34%)
	More than $100,000 a year	6 (8%)
Religious affiliation	Protestant Christian	25 (31%)
	Roman Catholic	10 (13%)
	Jewish	1 (1%)
	Wiccan or Pagan	7 (9%)
	Other (UU, Cherokee, Sufi, Hindu)	8 (10%)
	None	29 (36%)
Years belly dancing	Less than one year	17 (21%)
	One to less than five years	28 (35%)
	Five to less than ten years	15 (19%)
	Ten to less than twenty years	9 (11%)
	Twenty or more years	12 (15%)
Workplace gender	All/almost all women	19 (26%)
	Mostly women	19 (26%)
	Half men and half women	15 (21%)
	Mostly men	12 (17%)
	Almost all men	7 (10%)

The vast majority of the respondents are in school or are working in a variety of occupations. A little more than half of the sample work with primarily women in their places of business, while the other half of the sample is split between a balanced workplace gender composition and career settings that are dominated by men. Examples of the academic and professional fields represented in this sample include social work and counseling, computer programming and development, business, accounting, mathematics, veterinary medicine, health and medical, education, physical sciences (biology, chemistry, etc.), and full-time belly dance instructor and performer.

In addition to the information provided in the table, most of the participants have a background in other dance forms, such as ballet or jazz. The vast majority of dancers prefer the cabaret and tribal styles of belly dance. Forty-four express a preference for cabaret, while twenty prefer tribal belly dance. Nine dancers prefer folk styles, and five prefer fusion. All respondents have taken classes and dance in their homes. Fifty-six dancers have danced at haflas and workshops. Sixty-seven of the dancers have performed in public.

Protecting dancers' identities

The vast majority of dancers with whom I spoke gave me permission to use their actual names. However, I maintain confidentiality of their identities because (1) our professional protocol calls for confidentiality and (2) my participants and I can never completely anticipate how readers will react to the material in this book, and I want to protect my subjects from any unanticipated issues. Therefore, I use pseudonyms, change potentially identifying details, delete troupe names, and conceal locations throughout the book.

The discussion of stage names in Chapter 6 is one exception. I disclose actual dance names with all subjects' permission. Sharing dance names gives the reader a sense of the types of names some dancers elect to use in their respective dance communities and elsewhere. However, not all dancers discussed in this section participated in the formal data collection process, and due to the volume of interviews, many dancers with whom I spoke are not mentioned in this part of the book.

In many cases, informal conversations are also included with participants' permission. When obtaining expressed permission was not possible, additional details have been changed or omitted to further protect dancers' identities. I do not doubt that some dancers may identify themselves or others within the pages of this book. My hope is that their experiences are presented fairly and in ways that will not cause harm to themselves or disrupt their relationships within or outside belly dance communities.

Data analysis

The analyses are guided by both grounded theory (Charmaz 2014) and situational analysis (Clarke 2012). Both grounded theory and situational analysis are analytical processes that are rooted in the people who conduct them. As researchers, our backgrounds, experiences, and perspectives (both personal and academic) guide what we study and what we see to varying degrees (Charmaz 2014). The researcher's location and position is meaningful and produces one reflexive account of a study site (Charmaz 2014; Clarke 2012). In grounded theory, what we offer is our interpretation of our participants and their worlds rather than discovering some objective reality (Charmaz 2014). The stories I present here are certainly not the only stories to be told about the world of American belly dance. My position as a student and professional troupe member of (most recently) primarily improvisational tribal style and American Tribal Style belly dance privies me to a particular set of experiences and interactions that undoubtedly varies from someone who is not a performing troupe member, earns his or her living through belly dance, or someone immersed in one of the many tribal fusion or nightclub styles of dance. My troupe member status gives me a perspective, raises questions, and facilitates interactions with other dancers and troupe leaders, which sensitizes me to my broader data. Because of my troupe membership, I attended workshops and performances that I may not have done otherwise, and that provided important starting points for me to consider and sparked certain lines of inquiry to revisit in my data. Because my vantage point offers a particular set of experiences and interactions, other scholars and/or belly dancers have unique experiences and perspectives that will lead them to write a different book.

In situational analysis, a variety of elements, such as people, discourses, organizations, symbols, and institutions, both shape what occurs and are shaped by the actors within the situation. Therefore, situational analysis foregrounds the complex nature and messiness of life situations. We live in an age full of politics, images, and different identities (gendered, religious, and subcultural). We need to be sensitive to all of these various elements because they influence the people we study (Clarke and Friese 2007). Situational analysis focuses on identifying diversity, variation, complexity, and nuances within situations and social worlds (Clarke 2003, 2012).

Following and extending Strauss's (1978) work on social worlds, Clarke (1998) argues that focusing on the entirety of human and non-human elements that operate within a particular community allows us to examine diversity within social worlds to avoid presenting their inhabitants as monolithic. Both individual and collective identities are constructed through commitment to these worlds (Clarke 2006). Social worlds are interactive units that defy specific geographical boundaries, and they usually include segments and sub-divisions (Clarke 2006). Because of the potential vastness and complexity of social worlds, various arenas influence and are influenced by the world we study (Clarke 2006). It is precisely because these worlds are potentially so vast and include so many different elements that differences and conflict can arise. Persuasion, education, and repositioning are various strategies to deal with divisions (Clarke 2006).

Following Clarke's (2003, 2006, 2012) call for situational analyses of social worlds, I do not focus on just one aspect of belly dance. I pay attention to individuals, collectivities (typically in the form of troupes), relevant belly dance organizations, socio-cultural and symbolic elements (gender), physical spaces and areas that can shape experiences (classrooms and different performance venues), and a variety of discourses (normative expectations of dancers them-selves, cultural messages received from the media, and popular social ideas) to shed light on a variety of aspects within the world of belly dance. Simply perusing the various chapters in this book highlights a variety of characteristics and influences that I considered for this project.

Survey data from the brief questionnaires were entered into SPSS and were used to calculate frequencies describing the sample. They were primarily used to provide demographic and background information about the dancers and provide some context for their experiences. Interview transcriptions were imported into NVivo (a computer program that aids in the organization and analysis of qualitative data) and coded by me.

Grounded theory coding is a multi-stage process. First, codes are applied to each segment of data during a close and thorough reading of the data. This first stage of coding remains very close to the data. The goal is to ensure that the codes fit and are relevant to the world they describe as opposed to preconceived hypotheses generated in other forms of research (Charmaz 2014; Clarke 2012; Glaser and Strauss 1967). I applied codes to the data using phrases explicitly mentioned in those data. Rather than always using line-by-line coding, I coded larger chunks of data as part of incident-by-incident coding, which is particularly appropriate for ethnography (Charmaz 2014; Glaser 2001). Grounded theorists sometimes use "in vivo" codes that are spe-cial terms or language that respondents use themselves and are particularly meaningful for the world we are studying (Charmaz 2014). For instance, I did not create the language of "sisterhood" in Chapter 4. This language is embed-ded in the world of belly dance, and substantively important for many female participants.

Second, focused coding allows the researcher to synthesize the most signifi-cant and/or frequent codes to form broader themes (Charmaz 2014). While codes were combined, the data assigned those codes were checked against each other to ensure they were similar. The "constant comparative method" refers to continuously revisiting codes and themes to ensure they fit the data (Boeije 2002; Charmaz 2014; Glaser and Strauss 1967). I consulted various symbolic interaction literatures and other scholarly work for potential themes and constantly revisited existing literature throughout the writing of this book. I continuously examined the data with these themes in mind. I also remained open to new themes emerging during the analysis. The integration of codes and categories form the basis of a grounded theory and the majority of the data presentation within these pages (Charmaz 2014; Clarke 2012).

References

Aalten, Anna. 2004. "The Moment When It All Comes Together: Embodied Experiences in Ballet." *European Journal of Women's Studies* 11(3):263–276.

Abell, Steven C. and Maryse H. Richards. 1996. "The Relationship between Body Shape Satisfaction and Self-Esteem: An Investigation of Gender and Class Differences." *Journal of Youth and Adolescence* 25(5):691–703.

Albrecht, Stan L., Maria Cornwall, and Perry H. Cunningham. 1988. "Religious Leave-Taking: Disengagement and Disaffiliation among Mormons." pp. 62–80 in *Falling from the Faith: Causes and Consequences of Religious Apostasy*, ed. D. G. Bromley. Newbury Park, CA: Sage.

Albright, Ann Cooper. 1997. *Choreographing Difference: The Body and Identity in Contemporary Dance*. Hanover, NH: Wesleyan University Press.

Aleman, Ana M. Martinez. 2010. "College Women's Female Friendships: A Longitudinal View." *Journal of Higher Education* 81(5):553–582.

Al-Rawi, Rosina-Fawzia. 1999. *Grandmother's Secrets: The Ancient Rituals and Healing Power of Belly Dancing*. Brooklyn, NY: Interlink Books.

Altheide, David L. and Erdwin H. Pfuhl Jr. 1980. "Self-Accomplishment through Running." *Symbolic Interaction* 3(2):127–144.

Al Zayer, Penni. 2004. *Middle Eastern Dance*. Philadelphia, PA: Chelsea House Publishers.

Ammerman, Nancy T. 1987. *Bible Believers*. New Brunswick, NJ: Rutgers University Press.

Ammerman, Nancy T. 2007. "Introduction." pp. 3–18 in *Everyday Religion: Observing Modern Lives*, ed. N. Ammerman. New York: Oxford University Press.

Ammerman, Nancy T. 2010. "The Challenges of Pluralism: Locating Religion in a World of Diversity." *Social Compass* 57(2):154–167.

Ammerman, Nancy T. 2013. "Spiritual but Not Religious? Beyond Binary Choices in the Study of Religion." *Journal for the Scientific Study of Religion* 52(2): 258–278.

Anderson, Leon. 2006. "Analytic Autoethnography." *Journal of Contemporary Ethnography* 35(4):373–395.

Anderson, Leon and Jimmy D. Taylor. 2010. "Standing Out While Fitting In: Serious Leisure Identities and Aligning Actions among Skydivers and Gun Collectors." *Journal of Contemporary Ethnography* 39(1):34–59.

Archer, Larissa. 2013. "Bellydancing and Hummus: Third Fridays at Tannourine." *Huffington Post*. April 19.

Aries, Elizabeth J. and Fern L. Johnson. 1983. "Close Friendship in Adulthood: Conversational Content between Same Sex Friends." *Sex Roles* 9(12):1183–1196.

Atkins-Sayre, Wendy. 2005. "Naming Women: The Emergence of 'Ms.' as a Liberatory Title." *Women and Language* 28(1):8–16.

Atkinson, Paul. 2006. "Opera and the Embodiment of Performance." pp. 95–107 in *Body/Embodiment: Symbolic Interaction and the Sociology of the Body*, ed. Dennis Waskul and Phillip Vannini. Aldershot: Ashgate.

Aukett, Richard, Jane Ritchie, and Kathryn Mill. 1988. "Gender Differences in Friendship Patterns." *Sex Roles* 19(10):57–66.

Baldwin, Cheryl and Patricia Norris. 1999. "Exploring the Dimensions of Serious Leisure: 'Love me–Love my dog!'" *Journal of Leisure Research* 31(1):4–11.

Barkan, Ruth. 2004. *Nudity: A Cultural Anatomy*. Oxford: Berg.

Bartky, Sandra L. 1990. *Femininity and Domination: Studies in the Phenomenology of Oppression*. London: Routledge.

Bearman, Steve, Neill Korobov, and Avril Thorne. 2009. "The Fabric of Internalized Sexism." *Journal of Integrated Social Sciences* 1(1):10–47.

Beausoleil, Natalie. 1994. "Makeup in Everyday Life: An Inquiry into the Practices of Urban American Women of Diverse Backgrounds." pp. 33–57 in *Many Mirrors: Body Image and Social Relations*, ed. N. Sault. New Brunswick, NJ: Rutgers University Press.

Beck, Giles and Gordon Lynch. 2009. "'We Are All One, We Are All Gods': Negotiating Spirituality in the Conscious Partying Movement." *Journal of Contemporary Religion* 24(3):339–355.

Becker, Howard S. 2001. "Art as Collective Action." pp. 67–79 in *Popular Culture: Production and Consumption*, ed. C. Lee Harrington and Denise D. Bielby. Malden, MA: Blackwell.

Belly Dance Classes in the United States. 2014. Retrieved October 15, 2014 from http://us.bellydanceclasses.net/.

Bemiller, Michelle. 2005. "Men Who Cheer." *Sociological Focus* 38(3):205–222.

Bender, Courtney. 2010. *The New Metaphysicals: Spirituality and the American Religious Imagination*. Chicago, IL: University of Chicago Press.

Bernard, Jessie. 1981. *The Female World*. New York: Free Press.

Blumer, Herbert. 1969. *Symbolic Interactionism: Perspective and Method*. Englewood Cliffs, NJ: Prentice-Hall.

Bock, Sheila M. 2005. "From Harem Fantasy to Female Empowerment: Rhetorical Strategies and Dynamics of Style in American Belly Dance" (unpublished Master's thesis). Ohio State University, Columbus, Ohio.

Boeije, Hennie. 2002. "A Purposeful Approach to the Constant Comparative Method in the Analysis of Qualitative Interviews." *Quality and Quantity* 36(4):391–409.

Bordo, Susan. 2003. *Unbearable Weight: Feminism, Western Culture and the Body*. Los Angeles: University of California Press.

Bourdieu, Pierre. 2007 [1984]. *Distinction: A Social Critique of the Judgment of Taste*, trans. Richard Nice. Cambridge, MA: Harvard University Press.

Brown, Lyn M. 2003. *Girlfighting: Betrayal and Rejection among Girls*. New York: New York University Press.

Brown, Penelope and Stephen C. Levinson. 1987. *Politeness: Some Universals in Language*. Cambridge: Cambridge University Press.

Browning, Barbara. 1995. *Samba: Resistance in Motion*. Bloomington, IN: Indiana University Press.

Buchbinder, David. 2013. *Studying Men and Masculinities*. New York: Routledge.

Burke, Peter J. 2003. *Advances in Identity Theory and Research*. New York: Kluwer Academic/Plenum Publishers.

Burke, Peter J. and Jan E. Stets. 2009. *Identity Theory*. New York: Oxford University Press.

Burns, T. 1992. *Erving Goffman*. London: Routledge.

Burt, Ramsay. "The Performance of Unmarked Masculinity." pp. 150–167 in *When Men Dance: Choreographing Masculinities across Borders*, ed. Jennifer Fisher and Anthony Shay. New York: Oxford University Press.

Butler, Judith. 1988. "Performative Acts and Gender Constitution: An Essay in Phenomenology and Feminist Theory." *Theatre Journal* 40(4):519–531.

Butler, Judith. 1990. *Gender Trouble: Feminism and the Subversion of Identity*. New York: Routledge.

Cahill, Spencer E. and Robin Eggleston. 1995. "Reconsidering the Stigma of Physical Disability: Wheelchair Use and Public Kindness." *Sociological Quarterly* 36(4):681–698.

Carlton, Donna. 1994. *Looking for Little Egypt*. Bloomington, IN: IDD Books.

Carpentier, Joelle, Genevieve A. Mageau, and Robert J. Vallerand. 2012. "Ruminations and Flow: Why do People with a More Harmonious Passion Experience Higher Well-Being?" *Journal of Happiness Studies* 13(3):501–518.

Chaney, David. 2004. "Fragmented Culture and Subcultures." pp. 36–48 in *After Subculture: Critical Studies in Contemporary Youth Culture*, ed. A. Bennett and K. Kahn-Harris. New York: Palgrave Macmillan.

Charmaz, Kathy. 2002. "Qualitative Interviewing and Grounded Theory Analysis." pp. 675–693 in *Handbook for Interview Research: Context and Method*, ed. J. F. Grubrium and J. A. Holstein. Thousand Oaks, CA: Sage.

Charmaz, Kathy. 2009. "Shifting the Grounds: Constructivist Grounded Theory Methods." pp. 127–154 in *Developing Grounded Theory: The Second Generation*, ed. J. M. Morse, P. Noerager Stern, J. Corbin, B. Bowers, K. Charmaz, and A. E. Clarke. Walnut Creek, CA: Left Coast Press.

Charmaz, Kathy. 2014. *Constructing Grounded Theory*, 2nd edn. London: Sage.

Charmaz, Kathy and Dana Rosenfeld. 2006. "Reflections of the Body, Images of Self: Visibility and Invisibility in Chronic Illness and Disability." pp. 35–49 in *Body/Embodiment: Symbolic Interaction and the Sociology of the Body*, ed. Dennis Waskul and Phillip Vannini. Aldershot: Ashgate.

Chesler, Phyllis. 2001. *Woman's Inhumanity to Woman*. New York: Thunder's Mouth Press.

Chimot, Caroline and Catherine Louveau. 2010. "Becoming a Man While Playing a Female Sport: The Construction of Masculine Identity in Boys Doing Rhythmic Gymnastics." *International Review for the Sociology of Sport* 45(4):436–456.

Chrisler, Joan C. and Jean M. Lamont. 2002. "Can Exercise Contribute to the Goals of Feminist Therapy?" *Women & Therapy* 25(2):9–22.

Christ, Carol P. 1987. "Why Women Need the Goddess." pp. 117–132 in *Laughter of Aphrodite: Reflections on a Journey to the Goddess*, ed. C. P. Christ. San Francisco, CA: Harper.

Cimino, Richard and Don Lattin. 2002. *Shopping for Faith: American Religion in the New Millennium*. New York: Jossey-Bass.

Clarke, Adele E. 1998. *Disciplining Reproduction: Modernity, American Life Sciences, and the Problems of Sex*. Berkeley, CA: University of California Press.

Clarke, Adele E. 2003. "Situational Analysis: Grounded Theory Mapping After the Postmodern Turn." *Symbolic Interaction* 26(4):553–576.

Clarke, Adele E. 2006. "Social Worlds." pp. 4547–4549 in *Blackwell Encyclopedia of Sociology*, ed. G. Ritzer. Malden, MA: Wiley-Blackwell.

Clarke, Adele E. 2012. "Feminism, Grounded Theory, and Situational Analysis Revisited." pp. 388–412 in *Handbook of Feminist Research: Theory and Praxis*, ed. S. N. Hesse-Biber. Thousand Oaks, CA: Sage.

Clarke, Adele E. and Carrie Friese. 2007. "Grounded Theorizing Using Situational Analysis." pp. 363–397 in *The SAGE Handbook of Grounded Theory*, ed. A. Bryant and K. Charmaz. Thousand Oaks, CA: Sage.

Clarke, Laura H. 2011. *Facing Age: Women Growing Older in Anti-Aging Culture*. Lanham, MD: Rowman & Littlefield.

Clarke, Laura H. and Meridith Griffin. 2007. "The Body Natural and the Body Unnatural: Beauty Work and Aging." *Journal of Aging Studies* 21(3):187–201.

Clarke, Laura H. and Meridith Griffin. 2008. "Body Image and Aging: Older Women and the Embodiment of Trauma." *Women's Studies International Forum* 31(3):200–208.

Coates, Jennifer. 1996. *Women Talk*. Hoboken, NJ: Wiley-Blackwell.

Cohen, Stanley and Laurie Taylor. 1992. *Escape Attempts: The Theory and Practice of Resistance to Everyday Life*, 2nd edn. London: Routledge.

Comas-Diaz, Lillian and Marcella Bakur Weiner. 2013. "Sisters of the Heart: How Women's Friendships Heal." *Women & Therapy* 36(1):1–10.

Connell, Raewyn W. 1987. *Gender and Power: Society, the Person, and Sexuality Politics*. Stanford, CA: Stanford University Press.

Connell, Raewyn W. 2002. *Gender*. Malden, MA: Polity Press.

Connell, Raewyn W. 2005. "Globalization, Imperialism, and Masculinities." pp. 71–89 in *Handbook of Studies on Men and Masculinities*, ed. Michael S. Kimmel, Jeff Hearn, and R. W. Connell. Thousand Oaks, CA: Sage.

Cooley, Charles H. 1922. *Human Nature and the Social Order*. New York: Charles Scribner's Sons.

Cooley, Charles H. 1983 [1902]. *Human Nature and the Social Order*. Piscataway, NJ: Transaction.

Correll, Shelley and Cecilia Ridgeway. 2003. "Expectation States Theory." pp. 29–51 in *Handbook of Social Psychology*, ed. John DeLamater. New York: Springer.

Crawford, Robert. 1980. "Healthism and the Medicalization of Everyday Life." *International Journal of Health Services* 10(3):365–388.

Crick, Nicki R., Juan F. Casas, and David A. Nelson. 2002. "Toward a More Comprehensive Understanding of Peer Maltreatment: Studies of Relational Victimization." *Current Directions in Psychological Science* 11(3):98–101.

Crosby, Janice. 2000. "The Goddess Dances: Spirituality and American Women's Interpretations of Middle Eastern Dance." pp. 166–182 in *Daughters of the Goddess: Studies of Healing, Identity, and Empowerment*, ed. W. Griffin. Lanham, MD: AltaMira Press.

Crossley, Nick. 2005. "Mapping Reflexive Body Techniques: On Body Modification and Maintenance." *Body & Society* 11(1):1–35.

Crossley, Nick. 2006a. "In the Gym: Motives, Meaning, and Moral Careers." *Body & Society* 12(3):23–50.

Crossley, Nick. 2006b. "The Networked Body and the Question of Reflexivity." pp. 21–33 in *Body/Embodiment: Symbolic Interaction and the Sociology of the Body*, ed. D. Waskul and P. Vannini. Aldershot: Ashgate.

Crossley, Nick. 2006c. *Reflexive Embodiment in Contemporary Society*. Maidenhead: Open University Press.

Crothers, Laura M., Julaine E. Field, and Jered B. Kolbert. 2005. "Navigating Power, Control, and Being Nice: Aggression in Adolescent Girls' Friendships." *Journal of Counseling and Development* 83(3):349–354.

Csikszentmihalyi, Mihaly and Jeremy Hunter. 2003. "Happiness in Everyday Life: The Uses of Experience Sampling." *Journal of Happiness Studies* 4(2):185–199.

Dallal, Tamalyn. 2004. *Belly Dancing for Fitness: The Ultimate Dance Workout That Unleashes Your Creative Spirit*. Berkeley, CA: Ulysses Press.

Dellasega, Cheryl. 2005. *Mean Girls Grown Up: Adult Women Who Are Still Queen Bees, Middle Bees, and Afraid-To-Bees*. Hoboken, NJ: John Wiley.

D'Emilio, John and Estelle B. Freedman. 1997. *Intimate Matters: A History of Sexuality in America*, 2nd edn. Chicago, IL: University of Chicago Press.

Dennis, Alex and Peter J. Martin. 2005. "Symbolic Interactionism and the Concept of Power." *British Journal of Sociology* 56(2):191–213.

DeNora, Tia. 2000. *Music in Everyday Life*. Cambridge: Cambridge University Press.

Dilley, Rachel E. and Sheila J. Scraton. 2010. "Women, Climbing, and Serious Leisure." *Leisure Studies* 29(2):125–141.

Dolphina. 2005. *Bellydance: Get Fit and Feel Fabulous with the Unique Workout for the Mind and Body*. New York: DK Publishing.

Dox, Donnalee. 2005. "Spirit from the Body: Belly Dance as a Spiritual Practice." pp. 303–340 in *Belly Dance: Orientalism, Transnationalism, and Harem Fantasy*, ed. A. Shay and B. Sellers-Young. Costa Mesa, CA: Mazda.

Dox, Donnalee. 2006. "Dancing around Orientalism." *The Drama Review* 50:52–71.

Dupont, Tyler. "From Core to Consumer: The Informal Hierarchy of the Skateboard Scene." *Journal of Contemporary Ethnography* 43(5):556–581.

Durkheim, Émile. 1995 [1912]. *The Elementary Forms of the Religious Life*, trans. Karen E. Fields. New York: Free Press.

Durkin, Keith F. and Clifton D. Bryant. 1999. "Propagandizing Pederasty: A Thematic Analysis of the On-line Exculpatory Accounts of Unrepentant Pedophiles." *Deviant Behavior* 20(2):103–127.

Edgley, Charles. 2006. "The Fit and Healthy Body: Consumer Narratives and the Management of Postmodern Corporeity." pp. 231–245 in *Body/Embodiment:*

Symbolic Interaction and the Sociology of the Body, ed. D. Waskul and P. Vannini. Aldershot: Ashgate.

El Masri, Gamila. 2010. "Dances Along the Nile Part One: Raqs Al Assaya." Retrieved January 15, 2010 from www.gildedserpent.com/art43/gamilaniledance1.htm.

Epstein, Cynthia Fuchs. 1992. "Tinkerbells and Pinups: The Construction and Reconstruction of Gender Boundaries at Work." pp. 232–256 in *Cultivating Differences: Symbolic Boundaries and the Making of Inequality*, ed. M. Lamont and M. Fournier. Chicago, IL: University of Chicago Press.

Ezzell, Matthew B. 2009. "'Barbie Dolls' on the Pitch: Identity Work, Defensive Othering, and Inequality in Women's Rugby." *Social Problems* 56(1):111–131.

Farhana, Princess. 2007. *A Student's Guide to Belly Dance Styles*. Zaghareet. March/April:27–28.

Felder, Stefan. 2006. "The Gender Longevity Gap: Explaining the Difference between Singles and Couples." *Journal of Population Economics* 19(3):543–557.

Ferguson, Ann. 2000. *Bad Boys: Public Schools in the Making of Black Masculinity*. Ann Arbor, MI: University of Michigan Press.

Fine, Gary Alan. 1979. "Small Groups and Culture Creation: The Idioculture of Little League Baseball Teams." *American Sociological Review* 44(5):733–745.

Fine, Gary Alan. 1987. *With the Boys: Little League Baseball and Preadolescent Culture*. Chicago, IL: University of Chicago Press.

Fine, Gary Alan. 2002. *Shared Fantasy: Role-Playing Games as Social Worlds*. Chicago, IL: University of Chicago Press.

Fine, Gary Alan. 2006. "Shopfloor Cultures: The Idioculture of Production in Operational Meteorology." *Sociological Quarterly* 47(1):1–19.

Fine, Gary Alan. 2012a. "Group Culture and the Interaction Order: Local Sociology on the Meso-Level." *Annual Review of Sociology* 38:159–179.

Fine, Gary Alan. 2012b. *Tiny Publics: A Theory of Group Action and Culture*. New York: Russell Sage Foundation.

Fisher, Jennifer. 2009. "Maverick Men in Ballet: Rethinking the 'Making it Macho' Strategy." pp. 31–48 in *When Men Dance: Choreographing Masculinities across Borders*, ed. J. Fisher and A. Shay. New York: Oxford University Press.

Fisher, Jennifer and Anthony Shay. 2009. "Introduction." pp. 3–27 in *When Men Dance: Choreographing Masculinities across Borders*, ed. J. Fisher and A. Shay. New York: Oxford University Press.

Flinn, Juliana. 1995. "American Country Dancing: A Religious Experience." *Journal of Popular Culture* 29(1):61–69.

Flory, Richard. 1996. "Maintaining 'Christian Manliness' and 'Christian Womanliness': Controlling Gender in Christian Colleges, 1925–1991." pp. 51–79 in *The Power of Gender in Religion*, ed. G. Weatherby and S. Farrell. New York: McGraw-Hill.

Flory, Richard. 2000. "Conclusion: Toward a Theory of Generation X Religion." pp. 231–249 in *Gen X Religion*, ed. R. W. Flory and D. E. Miller. New York: Routledge.

Foltz, Tanice. 2006. "Drumming and Re-enchantment: Creating Spiritual Community." pp. 131–146 in *Popular Spiritualities: The Politics of Contemporary Enchantment*, ed. L. Hume and K. Mcphillips. Aldershot: Ashgate.

Foucault, Michel. 1976. *The History of Sexuality, Volume 1: The Will to Knowledge.* London: Penguin.

Frank, Katherine. 1988. "The Production of Identity and the Negotiation of Intimacy in a Gentleman's Club." *Sexualities* 1(2):175–201.

Fredrickson, Barbara L. and Tomi-Ann Roberts. 1997. "Objectification Theory: Toward Understanding Women's Lived Experiences and Mental Health Risks." *Psychology of Women Quarterly* 21(2):173–206.

Freysinger, Valeria J. 1995. "The Dialectics of Leisure and the Development of Women and Men in Mid-life: An Interpretative Study." *Journal of Leisure Research* 27(1):61–84.

Fuller, Robert C. 2001. *Spiritual, But Not Religious: Understanding Unchurched America.* New York: Oxford University Press.

Glaser, Barney G. 2001. *The Grounded Theory Perspective: Conceptualization Contrasted with Description.* Mill Valley, VA: Sociology Press.

Glaser, Barney G. and Anselm L. Strauss. 1967. *The Discovery of Grounded Theory: Strategies for Qualitative Research.* Chicago, IL: Aldine Publishing.

Goffman, Erving. 1959. *The Presentation of Self in Everyday Life.* Garden City, NY: Doubleday.

Goffman, Erving. 1961. *Encounters.* Indianapolis, IN: Bobbs-Merrill.

Goffman, Erving. 1963. *Stigma: Notes on the Management of a Spoiled Identity.* New York: Prentice-Hall.

Goffman, Erving. 1967. *Interaction Ritual: Essays on Face to Face Behavior.* Chicago, IL: Aldine Publishing.

Goffman, Erving. 1974. *Frame Analysis: An Essay on the Organization of Experience.* New York: Harper & Row.

Goodwin, Marjorie Harness. 2002. "Exclusion in Girls' Peer Groups: Ethnographic Analysis of Language Practices on the Playground." *Human Development* 45(6): 392–415.

Green, Eileen. 1998. "Women Doing Friendship: An Analysis of Women's Leisure as a Site of Identity Construction, Empowerment and Resistance." *Leisure Studies* 17(3):171–185.

Griffith, R. Marie. 2004. *Born Again Bodies: Flesh and Spirit in American Christianity.* Berkeley, CA: University of California Press.

Grogan, Sarah. 2008. *Body Image: Understanding Body Dissatisfaction in Men, Women, and Children.* New York: Routledge.

Grubrium, Jaber and James Holstein. 2003. "The Everyday Visibility of the Aging Body." pp. 205–227 in *Aging Bodies: Images and Everyday Experience,* ed. C. A. Faircloth. Walnut Creek, CA: AltaMira Press.

Gurrentz, Benjamin T. 2014. "A Brotherhood of Believers: Religious Identity and Boundary-Work in a Christian Fraternity." *Sociology of Religion* 75(1):113–135.

Haenfler, Ross. 2006. *Straightedge: Hardcore Punk, Clean-Living Youth, and Social Change.* New Brunswick, NJ: Rutgers University Press.

Haenfler, Ross. 2010. *Goths, Gamers, Grrrls: Deviance and Youth Subcultures.* New York: Oxford University.

Hagedorn, Katherine J. 2001. *Divine Utterances: The Performance of Afro-Cuban Santeria.* Washington, DC: Smithsonian Institution Press.

Harkness, Geoff. 2012. "True School: Situational Authenticity in Chicago's Hip-Hop Underground." *Cultural Sociology* 6(3):283–298.

Harrison, Anthony Kwame. 2008. "Racial Authenticity in Rap Music and Hip Hop." *Sociology Compass* 2(6):1783–1800.

Hayam. 2015. "What Makes a Belly Dancer Beautiful?" August 5, 2015. Accessed August 20, 2015 from http://bellydanceatanysize.com/makes-belly-dancer-beautiful/.

Henley, Nancy. 1986. *Body Politics: Power, Sex, and Nonverbal Communication.* New York: Prentice-Hall.

Hesse-Biber, Sharlene. 2006. *Am I Thin Enough Yet? The Cult of Thinness and the Commercialization of Identity*, 2nd edn. Oxford: Oxford University Press.

Hobin, Tina. 2003. *Belly Dance: The Dance of Mother Earth.* London: Marion Boyars.

Hochschild, Arlie R. 1979. "Emotion Work, Feeling Rules, and Social Structure." *American Journal of Sociology* 85(3):551–575.

Holstein, Martha B. 2006. "On Being an Aging Woman." pp. 313–334 in *Age Matters: Re-aligning Feminist Thinking*, ed. T. M. Calasanti and K. F. Sleven. New York: Routledge.

hooks, bell. 1984. *Feminist Theory: From Margin to Center.* Boston, MA: South End Press.

Howard, Judith A. 2000. "Social Psychology of Identities." *Annual Review of Sociology* 26:367–393.

Hughes, Michael. 2000. "Country Music as Impression Management: A Meditation on Fabricating Authenticity." *Poetics* 28(3):185–205.

Hunt, Pamela M. 2008. "From Festies to Tourrats: Examining the Relationship between Jamband Subculture Involvement and Role Meanings." *Social Psychology Quarterly* 71(4):356–378.

Hunt, Stephen J. 2004. "Acting the Part: 'Living History' as a Serious Leisure Pursuit." *Leisure Studies* 23(4):387–403.

Hutson, Scott R. 2000. "The Rave: Spiritual Healing in Modern Western Subcultures." *Anthropological Quarterly* 73(1):35–49.

Irwin, Katherine. 2001. "Legitimating the First Tattoo: Moral Passage through Informal Interaction." *Symbolic Interaction* 24(1):49–73.

Jahal, Jasmin. 2001. "Folkloric Dances." Accessed April 24, 2015 from www.jasminja-hal.com/articles/01_06_folkloric.html.

Jarrar, Randa. 2014. "Why I Can't Stand White Belly Dancers: Whether They Know it or Not, White Women who Practice Belly Dance are Engaging in Appropriation." Retrieved March 6, 2014 from Alternet.org.

Jeffreys, Sheila. 2005. *Beauty and Misogyny: Harmful Cultural Practices in the West.* New York: Routledge.

Jones, Ian. 2000. "A Model of Serious Leisure Identification: The Case of Football Fandom." *Leisure Studies* 19(4):283–298.

Jones, Stephanie J. and Elyn M. Palmer. 2011. "Glass Ceilings and Catfights: Career Barriers for Professional Women in Academia." *Advancing Women in Leadership* 31(1):189–198.

Jorgensen, Jeana. 2006. "'Whether Its Coins, Fringe, or Just Stuff That's Sparkly': Aesthetics and Utility in a Tribal Fusion Belly Dance Troupe's Costumes." *Midwestern Folklore* 32(1/2):83–97.

Jorgensen, Jeana. 2012. "Dancing the Numinous: Sacred and Spiritual Techniques of Contemporary American Belly Dancers." *Journal of Ethnology and Folkloristics* 6(2):3–28.

Karayanni, Stavros Stavrou. 2009. "Native Motion and Imperial Emotion: Male Performers of the 'Orient' and the Politics of the Imperial Gaze." pp. 314–348 in *When Men Dance: Choreographing Masculinities across Borders*, ed. J. Fisher and A. Shay. New York: Oxford University Press.

Kenny, Erin. 2007. "Bellydance in the Town Square: Leaking Peace through Tribal Style Identity." *Western Folklore* 66(3):301–327.

Khanolkar, Preeti R. and Paul D. McLean. 2012. "100-Percenting It: Videogame Play through the Eyes of Devoted Gamers." *Sociological Forum* 27(4):961–985.

Kilbourne, Jean. 1994. "Still Killing Us Softly: Advertising and the Obsession with Thinness." pp. 395–418 in *Feminist Perspectives on Eating Disorders*, ed. P. Fallon, M. A. Katzman, and S. C. Wooley. New York: Guilford Press.

Kimmel, Michael S. 2005. "Globalization and Its Mal(e)contents: The Gendered Moral and Political Economy of Terrorism." pp. 414–431 in *Handbook of Studies on Men and Masculinities*, ed. M. S. Kimmel, J. Hearn, and R. W. Connell. Thousand Oaks, CA: Sage.

Kimmel, Michael S. 2008. *Guyland*. New York: HarperCollins.

Knickmeyer, Nicole, Kim Sexton, and Nancy Nishimura. 2002. "The Impact of Same-Sex Friendships on the Well-Being of Women: A Review of the Literature." *Women & Therapy* 25(1):37–59.

Kraus, Rachel. 2009. "Straddling the Sacred and Secular: Creating a Spiritual Experience through Belly Dance." *Sociological Spectrum* 29(5):598–625.

Kraus, Rachel. 2010a. "They Danced in the Bible: Identity Integration among Christian Women who Belly Dance." *Sociology of Religion* 71(4):457–482.

Kraus, Rachel. 2010b. "We Are Not Strippers": How Belly Dancers Manage a (Soft) Stigmatized Serious Leisure Activity." *Symbolic Interaction* 33(3):435–455.

Kraus, Rachel. 2013. "'I Really Don't Do It for the Spirituality': How Often Do Belly Dancers Infuse Artistic Leisure with Spiritual Meaning?" *Implicit Religion* 16(3):301–318.

Kraus, Rachel. 2014. "Transforming Spirituality in Artistic Leisure: How the Spiritual Meaning of Belly Dance Changes Over Time." *Journal for the Scientific Study of Religion* 53(3):459–478.

Lamont, Michele. 1992. *Money, Morals, and Manners: The Culture of the French and the American Upper-Middle Class*. Chicago, IL: University of Chicago Press.

Lamont, Michele and Virag Molnar. 2002. "The Study of Boundaries in the Social Sciences." *Annual Review of Sociology* 28:167–195.

Lamont, Matthew, Millicent Kennelly, and Brent Moyle. 2014. "Costs and Perseverance in Serious Leisure Careers." *Leisure Sciences* 36(2):144–160.

Lash, Scott. 1991. "Genealogy and the Body: Foucault/Deleuze/Nietzsche." pp. 256–80 in *The Body: Social Process and Cultural Theory*, ed. M. Featherstone, M. Hepworth, and B. S. Turner. Newbury Park, CA: Sage.

Le, C. N. 2009. "The 1965 Immigration Act." Asian-Nation: The Landscape of Asian America." Retrieved September 9, 2009 from www.asian-nation.org/1965-immigration-act.shtml.

Link, Bruce G. and Jo C. Phelan. 2001. "Conceptualizing Stigma." *American Review of Sociology* 27(1):363–385.

Lofland, John and Lyn H. Lofland. 1995. *Analyzing Social Settings*, 3rd edn. Belmont, CA: Wadsworth.

Lofland, John, David Snow, Leon Anderson, and Lyn H. Lofland. 2006. *Analyzing Social Settings: A Guide to Qualitative Observation and Analysis*, 4th edn. Belmont, CA: Wadsworth.

Loseke, Donileen R. 1987. "Lived Realities and the Construction of Social Problems: The Case of Wife Abuse." *Symbolic Interaction* 10(2):229–243.

Lynch, Gordon. 2006. "The Role of Popular Music in the Construction of Alternative Spiritual Identities and Ideologies. *Journal for the Scientific Study of Religion* 45(4):481–488.

McCall, George and Jerry L. Simmons. 1966. *Identities and Interactions*. New York: Free Press.

McGuire, Meredith B. 1988. *Ritual Healing in Suburban America*. New Brunswick, NJ: Rutgers University Press.

McGuire, Meredith B. 2003a. "Gendered Spiritualities". pp. 170–180 in *Challenging Religion*, ed. J. A. Beckford and J. T. Richardson. London: Routledge.

McGuire, Meredith B. 2003b. "Why Bodies Matter: A Sociological Reflection on Spirituality and Materiality." *Spiritus: A Journal of Christian Spirituality* 3(1):1–18.

McGuire, Meredith B. 2007. "Embodied Practices: Negotiation and Resistance." pp. 187–200 in *Everyday Religion: Observing Modern Lives*, ed. N. Ammerman. New York: Oxford University Press.

McGuire, Meredith B. 2008. *Lived Religion: Faith and Practice in Everyday Life*. New York: Oxford University Press.

McKay, Jim, Janin Mikosza, and Brett Hutchins. 2005. "'Gentlemen, the Lunchbox Has Landed': Representations of Masculinities and Men's Bodies in the Popular Media." pp. 270–288 in *Handbook of Studies on Men and Masculinities*, ed. Michael S. Kimmel, Jeff Hearn, and R. W. Connell. Thousand Oaks, CA: Sage.

McLaren, Lindsay and Diana Kuh. 2004. "Women's Body Dissatisfaction, Social Class, and Social Mobility." *Social Science and Medicine* 58(9):1575–1584.

McRobbie, Angela and Jenny Garber. 1976. "Girls and Subcultures: An Explanation." pp. 209–22 in *Resistance through Rituals*, ed. Stuart Hall and Tony Jefferson. London: Routledge.

Magliocco, Sabina. 2004. *Witching Culture: Folklore and Neo-Paganism in America*. Philadelphia, PA: University of Pennsylvania Press.

Marion, Jonathan S. 2008. *Ballroom: Culture and Costume in Competitive Dance*. Oxford: Berg.

Martin, Peter J. 2004. "Cultures, Subculture and Social Organization." pp. 21–35 in *After Subculture: Critical Studies in Contemporary Youth Culture*, ed. A. Bennett and K. Kahn-Harris. New York: Palgrave Macmillan.

Mead, George Herbert. 1934. *Mind, Self, and Society from the Standpoint of a Social Behaviorist*. Chicago, IL: University of Chicago Press.

Melamed, David. 2013. "Do Magnitudes of Difference on Status Characteristics Matter for Small Group Inequalities?" *Social Science Research* 42(1):217–229.

Meltzer, B. N. 2003. "Lying: Deception in Human Affairs." *International Journal of Sociology and Social Policy* 23(6/7):60–79.

Mennesson, Christine. 2009. "Being a Man in Dance: Socialization Modes and Gender Identities." *Sport in Society: Cultures, Commerce, Media, Politics* 12(2):174–195.

Merton, Robert K. 1957. "The Role-Set: Problems in Sociological Theory." *British Journal of Sociology* 8(2):106–120.

Moberg, David O. 2000. "What Most Needs the Attention of Religion Researchers in the Twenty-First Century?" *Research in the Social Scientific Study of Religion* 11:1–21.

Moe, Angela M. 2011. "Belly Dancing Mommas: Challenging Cultural Discourses of Maternity." pp. 88–98 in *Embodied Resistance: Challenging the Norms, Breaking the Rules*, ed. C. Bobel and S. Kwan. Nashville, TN: Vanderbilt University Press.

Moe, Angela M. 2012. "Beyond the Belly: An Appraisal of Middle Eastern Dance (a.k.a. Belly Dance) as Leisure." *Journal of Leisure Research* 44(2):201–233.

Moe, Angela M. 2014. "Sequins, Sass and Sisterhood: An Exploration of Older Women's Belly Dancing." *Journal of Women and Aging* 26(1):39–65.

Monaghan, Lee F. 2005. "Big Handsome Men, Bears, and Others: Virtual Constructions of 'Fat Male Embodiment.'" *Body and Society* 11(2):81–111.

Monteiro, Nicole and Diana Wall. 2011. "African Dance as Healing Modality throughout the Diaspora: The Use of Ritual and Movement to Work through Trauma." *Journal of Pan African Studies* 4(6):234–252.

Monty, Paul Eugene. 1986. "Serena, Ruth St. Denis, and the Evolution of Belly Dance in America (1876–1976)." Ph.D. dissertation, School of Education, Health, Nursing and Arts Professions. New York University, New York.

Mooney, Nan. 2005. *I Can't Believe She Did That!* New York: St. Martin's Press.

Murray, Samantha. 2004. "Locating Aesthetics: Sexing the Fat Woman." *Social Semiotics* 14(3):237–247.

Nelson, Timothy J. 1996. "Sacrifice of Praise: Emotion and Collective Participation in an African-American Worship Service." *Sociology of Religion* 57(4):379–396.

Nericcio, Carolena. 2004. *The Art of Belly Dance: A Fun and Fabulous Way to Get Fit.* New York: Barnes and Noble.

Nooney, Jennifer Elizabeth. 2006. "Keeping the Faith: Religious Transmission and Apostasy in Generation X." Ph.D. dissertation, College of Humanities and Social Sciences, North Carolina State University, Raleigh, NC.

Nowotny, Kathryn M., Jennifer L. Fackler, Gianncarlo Muschi, Carol Vargas, Lindsey Wilson, and Joseph A. Kotarba. 2010. "Established Latino Music Scenes: Sense of Place and the Challenge of Authenticity." *Studies in Symbolic Interaction* 35(1):29–50.

O'Conner, Pat. 1992. *Friendships between Women: A Critical Review.* New York: Guilford Press.

Pascoe, C. J. 2011. *Dude You're a Fag: Masculinity and Sexuality in High School.* Oakland, CA: University of California Press.

Pasko, Lisa. 2002. "Naked Power: The Practice of Stripping as a Confidence Game." *Sexualities* 5(1):49–66.

Raphael, Melissa. 2008. "Gender." pp. 181–199 in *Handbook of Religion and Emotion*, ed. J. Carrigan. Oxford: Oxford University Press.

Raymond, Janice G. 1986. *A Passion for Friends: Toward a Philosophy of Female Affection*. Boston, MA: Beacon Press.

Rees-Denis, Paulette. *Tribal Vision: A Celebration of Life through Tribal Belly Dance*. Portland, OR: Cultivator Press.

Regehr, Kaitlyn. 2012. "The Rise of Recreational Burlesque: Bumping and Grinding Towards Empowerment." *Sexuality and Culture* 16(2):134–157.

Richardson, Deborah S. 2005. "The Myth of Female Passivity: Thirty Years of Revelations about Female Aggression." *Psychology of Women Quarterly* 29(3):238–247.

Risner, Doug. 2009. "What We Know about Boys Who Dance: The Limitations of Contemporary Masculinity and Dance Education." pp. 57–77 in *When Men Dance: Choreographing Masculinities across Borders*, ed. J. Fisher and A. Shay. New York: Oxford University Press.

Ronai, Carol R. 1992. "Managing Aging in Young Adulthood: The 'Aging' Table Dancer." *Journal of Aging Studies* 6(4):307–317.

Ronai, Carol R. and Rabecca Cross. 1998. "Dancing with Identity: Narrative Resistance Strategies of Male and Female Stripteasers." *Deviant Behavior* 19(2):99–119.

Roof, Wade Clark. 1999. *Spiritual Marketplace: Baby Boomers and the Remaking of American Religion*. Princeton, NJ: Princeton University Press.

Roof, Wade Clark and William McKinney. 1987. *American Mainline Religion: Its Changing Shape and Future*. New Brunswick, NJ: Rutgers University Press.

Royce, Anya Peterson. 2002. *The Anthropology of Dance*. London: Dance Books.

Said, Edward W. 1978. *Orientalism*. New York: Pantheon Books.

Saleem. 2009. "Saleem." pp. 375–377 in *When Men Dance: Choreographing Masculinities across Borders*, ed. Jennifer Fisher and Anthony Shay. New York: Oxford University Press.

Salimpour, Jamila. 2009. "Gunfighters and Ghawazee." Retrieved September 9, 2009 from www.suhailainternational.com/Pages/Articles/gunfighters.html.

Salimpour, Suhalia. 2009. "Jamila Salimpour." Retrieved September 9, 2009 from www.suhailainternational.com/Jamila.php.

Salomonsen, Jone. 2002. *Enchanted Feminism: The Reclaiming Witches of San Francisco*. London: Routledge.

Salutin, Marilyn. 1971. "Stripper Morality." *Trans-action* 8(8):12–22.

Sandstrom, Kent L., Daniel D. Martin, and Gary A. Fine. 2009. *Symbols, Selves, and Social Reality: A Symbolic Interactionist Approach to Social Psychology and Sociology*, 3rd edn. New York: Oxford University Press.

Savigliano, Marta E. 1998. "From Wallflowers to Femmes Fatales: Tango and the Performance of Passionate Femininity." pp. 103–110 in *The Passion of Music and Dance: Body, Gender, and Sexuality*, ed. William Washabaugh. Oxford: Berg.

Schmidt, Christopher and Donna E. Little. 2007. "Qualitative Insights into Leisure as a Spiritual Experience." *Journal of Leisure Research* 39(2):222–247.

Schmidt, Laura Tempest. 2009. "Quick Overview of Gothic Belly Dance." Retrieved September 9, 2009 from www.gothicbellydance.com/defined/about.html.

Schrock, Douglas and Michael Schwalbe. 2009. "Men, Masculinity, and Manhood Acts." *Annual Review of Sociology* 35:277–295.

Schwalbe, Michael. 1996. *Unlocking the Iron Cage: The Men's Movement, Gender Politics, and American Culture.* New York: Oxford University Press.

Scott, Susie. 2005. "The Red, Shaking Fool: Dramaturgical Dilemmas in Shyness." *Symbolic Interaction* 28(1):91–110.

Scott, Susie. 2009. "Reclothing the Emperor: The Swimming Pool as a Negotiated Order." *Symbolic Interaction* 32(2):123–145.

Scott, Susie. 2010. "How to Look Good (Nearly) Naked: The Performative Regulation of the Swimmer's Body." *Body & Society* 16(2):143–168.

Scott, Susie. 2012. "Intimate Deception in Everyday Life." *Studies in Symbolic Interaction* 39:251–279.

Sellers-Young, Barbara. 1992. "Raks el Sharki: Transculturation of a Folk Form." *Journal of Popular Culture* 26(2):141–152.

Sellers-Young, Barbara. 2009. "Ibrahim Farrah: Dancer, Teacher, Choreographer, Publisher." pp. 355–374 in *When Men Dance: Choreographing Masculinities across Borders,* ed. J. Fisher and A. Shay. New York: Oxford University Press.

Sharif, Keti. 2004. *Bellydance: A Guide to Middle Eastern Dance, Its Music, Its Culture, and Costume.* Sydney: Allen & Unwin.

Shaw, Aaron. 2012. "Centralized and Decentralized Gatekeeping in an Open Online Collective." *Politics and Society* 40(3):349–388.

Shay, Anthony. 2005. "The Male Dancer in the Middle East and Central Asia." pp 51–83 in *Belly-Dance: Orientalism, Transnationalism, and Harem Fantasy,* ed. A. Shay and B. Sellers-Young. Costa Mesa, CA: Mazda Publishers.

Shay, Anthony. 2008. *Dancing Across Borders: The American Fascination with Exotic Dance Forms.* Jefferson, NC: McFarland & Company.

Shay, Anthony. 2009. "Choreographing Masculinity: Hypermasculine Dance Styles as Invented Tradition in Eygpt, Iran, and Uzbekistan." pp. 287–308 in *When Men Dance: Choreographing Masculinities across Borders,* ed. J. Fisher and A. Shay. New York: Oxford University Press.

Shay, Anthony and Barbara Sellers-Young. 2005. "Introduction." pp. 1–25 in *Belly Dance: Orientalism, Transnationalism, and Harem Fantasy,* ed. A. Shay and B. Sellers-Young. Costa Mesa, CA: Mazda Publishers.

Shira. 2000. "The Spiritual Connection." pp. 68–70 in *The Bellydance Book: Rediscovering the Oldest Dance,* ed. T. Richards. Concord: Backbeat Press.

Shira. 2014. "All About Belly Dancing." Retrieved September 9, 2014 from www.shira.net.

Shuruk, Samira. 2014. "Standard Belly Dance Rates by Region." Retrieved September 9, 2014 from www.samirashuruk.com/standardrateslist.html.

Simmel, Georg. 1949. "The Sociology of Sociability." Trans. Everett C. Hughes. *American Journal of Sociology* 55(3):254–261.

Simmel, Georg. 1971. *On Individuality and Social Forms,* ed. Donald N. Levine. Chicago, IL: University of Chicago Press.

Simmons, Rachel. 2011. *Odd Girl Out, Revised and Updated: The Hidden Culture of Aggression in Girls.* Boston, MA: Houghton Mifflin Harcourt.

Sointu, Eeva and Linda Woodhead. 2008. "Spirituality, Gender, and Expressive Selfhood." *Journal for the Scientific Study of Religion* 47(2):259–276.

Stalp, Marybeth C., M. Elise Radina, and Annette Lynch. 2008. "'We do it cuz its fun': Gendered Fun and Leisure for Midlife Women through Red Hat Society Membership." *Sociological Perspectives* 51(2):325–347.

Stanczak, Gregory C. 2006. *Engaged Spirituality: Social Change and American Religion.* Piscataway, NJ: Rutgers University Press.

Stanley, T. L. 2004. "Pop Culture: Belly Dancing Slinks into the Mainstream." *Advertising Age* 75(1):6.

Stebbins, Robert A. 1969. "Role Distance, Role Distance Behaviour and Jazz Musicians." *British Journal of Sociology* 20(4):406–415.

Stebbins, Robert A. 2001. "Serious Leisure." *Society* 38(4):53–57.

Stebbins, Robert A. 2011. "The Semiotic Self and Serious Leisure." *American Sociologist* 42(2–3):238–248.

Steensland, Brian, Jerry Z. Park, Mark D. Regnerus, Lynn D. Robinson, W. Bradford Wilcox, and Robert D. Woodberry. 2000. "The Measure of American Religion: Toward Improving the State of the Art." *Social Forces* 79(1):291–318.

Stephens, Neil and Sara Delamont. 2006. "Samba no Mar: Bodies, Movement and Idiom in *Capoeira*." pp. 109–122 in *Body/Embodiment: Symbolic Interaction and the Sociology of the Body,* ed. Dennis Waskul and Phillip Vannini. Aldershot: Ashgate.

Stewart, Iris J. 2000. *Sacred Women, Sacred Dance: Awakening Spirituality through Movement and Ritual.* Rochester: Inner Traditions.

Stolzenberg, Ross M., Mary Blair-Loy, and Linda J. Waite. 1995. "Religious Participation in Early Adulthood: Age and Family Life Cycle Effects on Church Membership." *American Sociological Review* 60(1):84–103.

Strauss, Anselm L. 1959. *Mirrors and Masks: The Search for Identity.* Glencoe, IL: Free Press.

Strauss, Anselm L. 1964. *George Herbert Mead on Social Psychology.* Chicago, IL: University of Chicago Press.

Strauss, Anselm L. 1978. "A Social Worlds Perspective." *Studies in Symbolic Interaction.* 1:119–128.

Striegel-Moore, Ruth H. and Debra L. Franko. 2002. "Body Image Issues among Girls and Women." pp. 183–191 in *Body Image: A Handbook of Theory, Research, and Clinical Practice,* ed. T. F. Cash and T. Pruzinsky. New York: Guilford Press.

Stryker, Sheldon. 1980. *Symbolic Interactionism: A Social Structural Version.* Menlo Park, CA: Benjamin Cummings.

Stryker, Sheldon and Peter J. Burke. 2000. "The Past, Present, and Future of an Identity Theory." *Social Psychology Quarterly* 63(4):284–297.

Stryker, Sheldon and Richard T. Serpe. 1994. "Identity Salience and Psychological Centrality: Equivalent, Overlapping, or Complementary Concepts?" *Social Psychology Quarterly* 57(1):16–35.

Swarts, Heidi. 2011. "Drawing New Symbolic Boundaries over Old Social Boundaries: Forging Social Movement Unity in Congregation-Based Community Organizing." *Sociological Perspectives* 54(3):453–477.

Tajfel, Henri and John C. Turner. 1986. "The Social Identity Theory of Intergroup Behavior." pp. 7–24 in *Psychology of Intergroup Relations*, ed. S. Worchel and W.G. Austin. Chicago, IL: Nelson.

195

Takahashi, Melanie and Tim Olaveson. 2003. "Music, Dance, and Raving Bodies: Raving as Spirituality in the Central Canadian Rave Scene." *Journal of Ritual Studies* 17(2):72–95.

Tanenbaum, Leora. 2000. *Slut! Growing Up Female with a Bad Reputation*. New York: Harper Perennial.

Tanenbaum, Leora. 2002. *Catfight: Rivalries among Women – From Diets to Dating, From the Boardroom to the Delivery Room*. New York: Harper Perennial.

Taylor, Charles. 2002. "Democracy, Inclusive and Exclusive." pp. 181–194 in *Meaning and Modernity: Religion, Polity, and the Self*, ed. R. Madsen, W. Sullivan, A. Swindler, and S. Tipton. Berkeley, CA: University of California Press.

Thomas, William I. and Dorothy Thomas. 1928. *The Child in America*. New York: Knopf.

Thompson, William E. and Jack L. Harred. 1992. "Topless Dancers: Managing Stigma in a Deviant Occupation." *Deviant Behavior* 13(3):291–311.

Thompson, William E., Jack L. Harred, and Barbara E. Burks. 2003. "Managing the Stigma of Topless Dancing: A Decade Later." *Deviant Behavior* 24(6):551–570.

Thorne, Barrie. 1993. *Gender Play: Girls and Boys in School*. New Brunswick, NJ: Rutgers University Press.

Tobin, Jeffrey. 1998. "Tango and the Scandal of Homosocial Desire." pp. 79–102 in *The Passion of Music and Dance: Body, Gender, and Sexuality*, ed. William Washabaugh. Oxford: Berg.

Tolman, Deborah L. 2002. *Dilemmas of Desire: Teenage Girls Talk about Sexuality*. Cambridge, MA: Harvard University Press.

Turner, Bryan. 1984. *The Body and Social Theory*. Thousand Oaks, CA: Sage.

Turner, Ralph H. 1956. "Role-Taking, Role Standpoint, and Reference-Group Behavior." *American Journal of Sociology* 61(4):316–328.

Turner, Ralph H. 1962. "Role-Taking: Process versus Conformity." pp. 20–40 in *Human Behavior and Social Processes*, ed. A. M. Rose. Boston, MA: Houghton Mifflin.

Turner, Ralph H. 1978. "The Role and the Person." *American Journal of Sociology* 84(1):1–23.

Unruh, David R. 1980. "The Nature of Social Worlds." *Pacific Sociological Review* 23:271–296.

van Nieuwkerk, Karin. 1995. *A Trade Like Any Other: Female Singers and Dancers in Egypt*. Austin, TX: University of Texas Press.

Vannini, Phillip and Dennis D. Waskul. 2006. "Body Ekstasis: Socio-Semiotic Reflections on Surpassing the Dualism of Body-Image." pp. 183–200 in *Body/Embodiment: Symbolic Interaction and the Sociology of the Body*, ed. Dennis Waskul and Phillip Vannini. Aldershot: Ashgate.

Vannini, Phillip and J. Patrick Williams. 2009. *Authenticity in Culture, Self, and Society*. Burlington, VT: Ashgate.

Viorst, Judith. 1998. *Necessary Losses: The Loves, Illusions, Dependencies, and Impossible Expectations that all of us Have to Give Up in Order to Grow Up*. New York: Free Press.

Wade, Lisa and Myra Marx Ferree. 2015. *Gender: Ideas, Interactions, Institutions*. New York: W. W. Norton.

Waskul, Dennis D. 2002. "The Naked Self: Being a Body in Televideo Cybersex." *Symbolic Interaction* 25(2):199–227.

Waskul, Dennis D. 2003. *Self-Games and Body-Play: Personhood in Online Chat and Cybersex*. New York: Peter Lang.

Waskul, Dennis and Matt Lust. 2004. "Role-Playing and Playing Roles: The Person, Player, and Persona in Fantasy Role-Playing." *Symbolic Interaction* 27(3):333–356.

Waskul, Dennis and Justin A. Martin. 2010. "Now the Orgy is Over." *Symbolic Interaction* 33(2):297–318.

Waskul, Dennis and Pamela van der Riet. 2002. "The Abject Embodiment of Cancer Patients: Dignity, Selfhood, and the Grotesque Body." *Symbolic Interaction* 25(4):487–513.

Waskul, Dennis D. and Phillip Vannini. 2006. "Introduction: The Body in Symbolic Interaction." pp. 1–18 in *Body/Embodiment: Symbolic Interaction and the Sociology of the Body*, ed. D. D. Waskul and P .Vannini. Aldershot: Ashgate.

Weber, Max. 1958. "The Three Types of Legitimate Rule." Trans. Hans Gerth. *Berkel Publications in Society and Institutions* 4(1):1–11.

Weinberg, Martin S. and Colin J. Williams. 2010. "Bare Bodies: Nudity, Gender, and the Looking Glass Body." *Sociological Forum* 25(1):47–67.

Weitz, Rose. 2001. "Women and their Hair: Seeking Power through Resistance and Accommodation." *Gender and Society* 15(5):667–686.

West, Candace and Don H. Zimmerman. 1987. "Doing Gender." *Gender and Society* 1(2):125–151.

Wilkins, Amy C. 2008. *Wannabes, Goths, and Christians: The Boundaries of Sex, Style, and Status*. Chicago, IL: University of Chicago Press.

Williams, Christine L. 1992. "The Glass Escalator: Hidden Advantages for Men in the 'Female' Professions." *Social Problems* 39(3):253–267.

Williams, Dorie Giles. 1985. "Gender, Masculinity-Femininity, and Emotional Intimacy in Same-Sex Friendship." *Sex Roles* 12(5):587–600.

Williams, J. Patrick. 2006. "Authentic Identities: Straightedge Subculture, Music, and the Internet." *Journal of Contemporary Ethnography* 35(2):173–200.

Williams, Roman R. 2010. "Space for God: Lived Religion at Work, Home and Play." *Sociology of Religion* 71(3):257–279.

Wolf, Naomi. 1990. *The Beauty Myth*. Toronto: Vintage Books.

Wood, Robert. 2003. "The Straightedge Youth Sub-Culture: Observations on the Complexity of Sub-Cultural Identity." *Journal of Youth Studies* 6(1):33–52.

Woodhead, Linda. 2002. "Women and Religion." pp. 332–356 in *Religion in the Modern World*, ed. L. Woodhead. London: Routledge.

Woods, Teresa and Gail Ironson. 1999. "Religion and Spirituality in the Face of Illness." *Journal of Health Psychology* 4(3):393–412.

Wulff, Helena. 1998. *Ballet across Borders: Career and Culture in the World of Dancers*. Oxford: Berg.

Wuthnow, Robert. 2001. *Creative Spirituality: The Way of the Artist*. Berkeley, CA: University of California Press.

Wuthnow, Robert. 2003. *All in Sync: How Music and Art are Revitalizing American Religion*. Berkeley, CA: University of California Press.

Xie, Hongling, Dylan J. Swift, Beverly D. Cairns, and Robert B. Cairns. 2002. "Aggressive Behaviors in Social Interaction and Developmental Adaptation:

A Narrative Analysis of Interpersonal Conflicts during Early Adolescence." *Social Development* 11(2):205–224.

Zenuba. 2000. "American Tribal Style Belly Dance." pp. 38–40 in *The Bellydance Book: Rediscovering the Oldest Dance*, ed. T. Richards. Concord: Backbeat.

Zinnbauer, Brian J. and Kenneth L. Pargament. 2005. "Religiousness and Spirituality." pp. 21–42 in *The Handbook of the Psychology of Religion and Spirituality*, ed. R. F. Paloutzian and C. L. Park. New York: Guilford Press.

Zinnbauer, Brian J., Kenneth I. Pargament, and Allie B. Scott. 1999. "The Emerging Meanings of Religiousness and Spirituality: Problems and Prospects." *Journal of Personality* 67(6):889–919.

Zuckerman, Phil. 2012. *Faith No More: Why People Reject Religion*. New York: Oxford University Press.

Index